EPA/600/R-02/044
March 2003
www.epa.gov/ncea

EPA Handbook for Use of Data from the National Health and Nutrition Examination Surveys (NHANES): A Goldmine of Data for Environmental Health Analyses

National Center for Environmental Assessment–Washington Office
Office of Research and Development
U.S. Environmental Protection Agency
Washington, DC 20460

DISCLAIMER

This document has been reviewed in accordance with U.S. Environmental Protection Agency policy and approved for publication. Mention of trade names or commercial products does not constitute endorsement or recommendation for use.

ABSTRACT

This Handbook provides descriptive background information and general guidance on how to access and use data from the National Health and Nutrition Examination Surveys (NHANES). This is an enormous human database that can be used to develop information suitable for use in risk assessments, and to support regulatory and policy needs of EPA. For more than 30 years, EPA has been one of many collaborating agencies that help plan and support funding of data collection through NHANES. Because only a limited number of Agency managers and staff are aware of the content and availability of this rich database, this Handbook was developed to familiarize staffs with NHANES and foster increased use of the data to support EPA needs. Despite the limitations and complex design of this survey, it is clear that NHANES is a unique, rich database that offers a tremendous amount of human health, nutrition, and exposure information, and will continue to do so into the future. It is hoped that by informing staff about NHANES, this Handbook will encourage efforts to "mine" the data to support Agency needs across the program offices. It is also hoped that innovative approaches (e.g., using geographic information systems; linking NHANES to available databases such as the National Death Index), will be developed to analyze the data in new ways that produce information that is useful to the mission of the Agency. Now that the National Center for Health Statistics (NCHS) has established their Research Data Center, it should be possible to conduct studies that were impossible in the past because of lack of access to sensitive data. Finally, more thought should be given to designing and conducting studies that make use of subjects' biological samples (blood, urine, saliva) stored by NCHS. These samples offer a rare opportunity to study potential biomarkers of exposure and/or effects on a national sample of the U.S. population and link the data to health, nutrition, exposure and socioeconomic data collected in the baseline surveys.

Preferred citation:
U.S. Environmental Protection Agency (EPA). (2003) Handbook for use of data from the national health and nutrition examination surveys (NHANES). National Center for Environmental Assessment, Washington, DC: EPA/600/R-02/044. Available from: National Technical Information Service, Springfield, VA, and <http://www.epa.gov/ncea>.

TABLE OF CONTENTS

TABLE OF CONTENTS (continued)

LIST OF TABLES

AUTHORS, CONTRIBUTORS, AND REVIEWERS

The National Center for Environmental Assessment–Washington Office within EPA's Office of Research and Development was responsible for the preparation of this Handbook.

AUTHOR
Susan Perlin
U.S. Environmental Protection Agency
National Center for Environmental Assessment-W
Washington, DC 20460

CONTRIBUTORS TO APPENDIX IX
Elmer Akin
U.S. Environmental Protection Agency Region 4,
Waste Management Div.
Atlanta, GA

Ruth Allen
U.S. Environmental Protection Agency
Office of Pesticide Programs
Office of Prevention, Pesticides and Toxic Substances
Washington, DC 20460

Denis Borum
U.S. Environmental Protection Agency
Office of Science and Technology
Office of Water
Washington, DC 20460

Rebecca Calderon
U.S. Environmental Protection Agency
Human Studies Division
National Health & Environmental Effects Research Lab
Research Triangle Park, NC

Robert Chapman
U.S. Environmental Protection Agency
National Center for Environmental Assessment-RTP
Research Triangle Park, NC

Chuck French
U.S. Environmental Protection Agency
Office of Air Quality Planning and Standards
Office of Air and Radiation
Research Triangle Park, NC

Elizabeth Hilborn
U.S. Environmental Protection Agency
Human Studies Division
National Health & Environmental Effects Research Lab
Research Triangle Park, NC

Helen Jacobs
U.S. Environmental Protection Agency
Office of Science and Technology
Office of Water
Washington, DC 20460

Thomas McCurdy
U.S. Environmental Protection Agency
National Exposure Research Laboratory
Research Triangle Park, NC

Ron Morony
U.S. Environmental Protection Agency
Office of Pollution, Prevention and Toxics
Office of Prevention, Pesticides and Toxic Substances
Washington, DC 20460

Jacqueline Moya
U.S. Environmental Protection Agency
National Center for Environmental Assessment-W
Washington, DC 20460

David Otto
U.S. Environmental Protection Agency
Human Studies Div.
Health & Environmental Effects Research Lab
Research Triangle Park, NC

James Quackenboss
U.S. Environmental Protection Agency
National Exposure Research Laboratory
Office of Research and Development
Las Vegas, NV

AUTHORS, CONTRIBUTORS, AND REVIEWERS (continued)

Dina Schreinemachers
U.S. Environmental Protection Agency
Human Studies Division
National Health & Environmental Effects Research Lab
Research Triangle Park, NC

Brad Schultz
U.S. Environmental Protection Agency
Office of Pollution, Prevention and Toxics
Office of Prevention, Pesticides and Toxic Substances
Washington, DC 20460

John Schwemberger
U.S. Environmental Protection Agency
Office of Pollution, Prevention and Toxics
Office of Prevention, Pesticides and Toxic Substances
Washington, DC 20460

Sherry Selevan
U.S. Environmental Protection Agency
National Center for Environmental Assessment-W
Washington, DC 20460

Marc Stifelman
U.S. Environmental Protection Agency, Region 10
Office of Environmental Assessment
Seattle, WA

Amina Wilkins
U.S. Environmental Protection Agency
National Center for Environmental Assessment-W
Washington, DC 20460

REVIEWERS

David Cleverly
U.S. Environmental Protection Agency
National Center for Environmental Assessment-W
Washington, DC 20460

Charles Dillon
National Center for Health Statistics
Hyattsville, MD 20782

Susan Schober
National Center for Health Statistics
Hyattsville, MD 20782

Wilbur Hadden
National Center for Health Statistics
Hyattsville, MD 20782

Sherry Selevan
U.S. Environmental Protection Agency
National Center for Environmental Assessment-W
Washington, DC 20460

ACRONYMS AND ABBREVIATIONS

BP- Blood pressure

Cd - Cadmium

CDC- Centers for Disease Control and Prevention

CNS- Central nervous system

CO - Carbon Monoxide. One of the six air pollutants the EPA regulates under NAAQS.

DEHLS - Division of Environmental Health Laboratory Sciences

DHHS - Department of Health and Human Services

EKG - Electrocardiogram

EPA - Environmental Protection Agency

FEV1 - Forced Expiratory Volume in the first second

FVC - Forced Vital Capacity

GIS - Geographical Information Systems

Hg - Mercury

HHANES - Hispanic Health and Nutrition Examination Survey

IRB - Institutional Review Board at NCHS

MEC - Mobile Examination Center

NAAQS- National Ambient Air Quality Standard pollutants, which include ozone, sulfur dioxide, nitrogen oxide, particulate matter, lead and carbon monoxide.

NCEA - National Center for Environmental Assessment. This is an EPA office.

NCEH - National Center for Environmental Health. This is a CDC lab.

NCHS - National Center for Health Statistics. This is a CDC office.

NDI - National Death Index

NH2MS- National Health and Nutrition Examination Survey-II Mortality Study

NHANES - National Health and Nutrition Examination Survey

NHDS - National Hospital Discharge Survey

NHEFS - NHANES Epidemiological Followup Study

NHES - National Health and Examination Survey

NHIS - National Health Interview Survey

NIOSH - National Institute of Occupational Safety and Health

NOx - Nitrogen oxides.

NSFG - National Survey of Family Growth

NTIS - National Technical Information Service

O3 - Ozone. One of the six air pollutants the EPA regulates under the NAAQS.

OGGT - Oral Glucose Tolerance Test

ORD - Office of Research and Development. This is an EPA office.

Pb - Lead. One of the six air pollutants the EPA regulates under the NAAQS.

PbB - Blood lead

PM10 - PM10 is defined as particulate matter (PM) with a mass median aerodynamic diameter less than 10 micrometers (um). One of the six air pollutants the EPA regulates under the NAAQS.

PSU - Primary Sampling Unit, usually a county

ACRONYMS AND ABBREVIATIONS (continued)

QA/QC - Quality Assurance/Quality Control
RDC- Research Data Center. This is a facility in NCHS.
SEQN - Sample Sequence Number. This is the unique identification number given to each
NHANES subject.
SES - Socioeconomic status
SOx - Sulfur oxides
SP - Sample Person in NHANES
USDA - U.S. Department of Agriculture
VOCs - Volatile organic compounds

1.0 PURPOSE OF THIS HANDBOOK

The U.S. Environmental Protection Agency's (EPA's) National Center for Environmental Assessment (NCEA), in the Office of Research and Development (ORD) has developed this Handbook to provide descriptive background information and general guidance on how to access and use data from the National Health and Nutrition Examination Surveys (NHANES). This is an enormous human database that can be used to develop information suitable for use in risk assessments, and to support regulatory and policy needs of EPA. For more than 30 years, EPA has been one of many collaborating agencies that help plan and support funding of data collection through NHANES. Because only a limited number of Agency managers and staff are aware of the content and availability of this rich database, NCEA developed this Handbook to familiarize staffs with NHANES and foster increased use of the data to support EPA needs. This Handbook will be disseminated throughout the Agency via the EPA intranet.

This Handbook is not be a treatise on how to conduct an epidemiology study using NHANES data. It is assumed that the audience is composed of epidemiologists, statisticians and analysts familiar with appropriate research methods and how to interpret the findings, but unfamiliar with the purpose, content, limitations and potential usefulness of NHANES for supporting Agency risk assessment, policy and regulatory needs. This Handbook will also be useful to EPA managers to provide them with an overview of the survey. This Handbook provides the following: purpose of the Handbook and the EPA NHANES Users Group (Sections 1.0 and 2.0); summary of the history and content of NHANES (Sections 3.0 and 4.0; Appendices II through VII); overview of how the surveys are conducted and how to obtain the data (Sections 3.0, 4.0 and 5.0); types of analyses that can be conducted with NHANES data and can support EPA risk assessment, policy and regulatory needs (Section 6.0; Appendices VIII and IX); availability and potential use of stored NHANES biological samples to support EPA needs (Section 7.0); discussion of the major limitations to use of NHANES data (i.e., can not perform local studies; issues of confidentiality) and some precautions on use and interpretation of study results (Section 8.0); discussion of issues with analysis of NHANES data, such as the need for weighting, and compensating for nonresponse bias (Section 9.0).

From this Handbook, the reader should gain a basic understanding of what data are available through NHANES; how to obtain the data; if the data are potentially suitable for supporting the needs of his/her office; key limitations of the data; and what types of analyses are possible. As indicated in Sections 3 and 6, and Appendices VIII and IX, NHANES data can be used to support a variety of environmental applications, such as: 1) evaluation of health effects associated with exposure to certain pollutants; 2) estimation of the levels of certain pollutants (e.g., lead, mercury, pesticides) in the general population based on chemical biomarkers in blood and/or urine; 3) establishment of population reference standards for various physiological parameters (e.g., height and weight, lung function) and; 4) examination of how personal risk factors (e.g., smoking, poor nutrition, obesity, poverty) interact with chemical exposures to affect health. Based on the information provided in the summaries of EPA studies that have used NHANES data (Appendix IX), the reader can also contact EPA scientists involved with specific studies to gain more insight into issues surrounding use of these data.

1

2.0. EPA NHANES USERS GROUP

EPA has an NHANES Users Group for anyone in the Agency who is interested in using the survey data. The Group has monthly conference calls where ideas are shared; members help each other with analytical problems; and everyone is kept apprized of issues and data collection activities of the on-going survey, NHANES99+. If you are interested in being included on the e-mail list and joining the Group, please contact Susan Perlin at perlin.susan@epa.gov.

3.0 OVERVIEW AND BACKGROUND OF NHANES

The National Center for Health Statistics (NCHS), which is part of the Centers for Disease Control and Prevention (CDC), has been collecting data on the health and nutrition status of the U.S. population for many decades. In 1956 the National Health Survey Act was passed, authorizing establishment of a continuous survey to provide current statistical data on the amount, distribution, and effects of illness and disability in the United States. Under this Act, data are to be obtained from at least three sources: personal interviews; clinical tests, measurements, and physical examinations; and from medical care facilities. Since passage of the Act, NCHS has conducted seven major surveys, resulting in extensive, publicly available databases containing varying amounts of information on health effects, nutrition, and environmental exposures from representative samples of the U.S. population. <http://www.cdc.gov/nchs/about/major/nhanes/history.htm>.

The National Health Examination Survey (NHES) was the first survey resulting from the Act. Within the first decade, three NHES surveys, each with approximately 7,500 subjects, were conducted:

NHES I: (1960-62). Focused on selected chronic diseases of adults 18 to 79 years old.
NHES II: (1963-65). Focused on growth and development of children 6 to11 years old.
NHES III: (1966-70). Focused on growth and development of children 12 to17 years old.

In the 1970s, with the discovery of the link between nutrition and certain diseases, the NHES was expanded to include collection of nutritional information, and the name of the survey was changed to the National Health and Nutrition Examination Survey (NHANES) to reflect this expansion. The EPA is one of many federal agencies that collaborates with NCHS to support NHANES. Other collaborating agencies include: Centers for Disease Control and Prevention, Food and Drug Administration, National Institutes of Health, National Institutes of Mental Health, National Institute for Environmental Health Sciences, Health Resources and Services Administration, Agency for Toxic Substances and Disease Registry, National Institute of Occupational Safety and Health, and the Social Security Administration.

In addition to the NHES and NHANES, NCHS also collects human data through a variety of other surveys, including the National Health Interview Survey (NHIS), the Survey of Family Growth (NSFG), National Hospital Discharge Survey, and the National Death Index (NDI). This Handbook pertains only to the NHANES surveys. For additional information on the history of NHANES, see <http://www.cdc.gov/nchs/about/major/nhanes/history.htm_>. For more information on other surveys conducted by NCHS, see <http://www.cdc.gov/nchs>.

Five major goals of NHANES are to provide the following:
1) national population reference distributions of selected health parameters (i.e., height, weight, cholesterol levels);
2) national prevalence data on diseases, functional impairment, and risk factors (i.e., heart disease, respiratory diseases, smoking, exposure to environmental pollutants);
3) information on secular changes in selected diseases and risk factors;
4) information to help understand disease etiology; and
5) information for investigating the natural history of selected diseases.

The last two goals of understanding disease etiology and the natural history of selected diseases are to be met through planned follow-up surveys of cohorts of initial respondents from each of the surveys (See Section 3.1) (NCHS, 1992b).

Since 1971 there have been four discrete NHANES (see Table 1). The latest survey, NHANES99+, went into the field in March 1999 and differs from the previous surveys in that it will collect annual data continuously into the future. Since NHANES will be in the field continuously, there is also a new naming convention to indicate the specific year of the survey (NHANES-99, NHANES-00, NHANES-01, etc.) When referring to the current NHANES in general, without reference to a specific year, it is called NHANES99+.

NHANES uses a complex, stratified, multistage, probability cluster design to select a representative sample of the noninstitutionalized, civilian U.S. population. A four-stage sample design is used, as follows: 1) Primary Sampling Units (PSUs) comprising mostly counties; 2) area segments within PSUs, 3) households within area segments, and 4) persons within households. It is beyond the scope of this Handbook to provide a detailed discussion of this complicated survey design. See Appendix I for information on the sample design of NHANES-III, which is similar to the design for all the NHANES. The reader also is referred to the following references for more complete discussions of the NHANES sample design: for NHANES-I, see NCHS (1973, 1977, 1978); for NHANES-II, see NCHS (1981); for HHANES see NCHS (1985); and for NHANES-III see NCHS (1994b, 1996c).

As noted in Table 1, each NHANES oversamples certain population subgroups. Oversampling is conducted for people in specific age/race/ethnicity/socioeconomic subgroups to help ensure there will be sufficient numbers of subjects to support valid analyses. The following excerpt from (NCHS, 1996c) helps to explain why there is a need to oversample certain subgroups:

"Older persons, children, Mexican-Americans, and black persons were oversampled in NHANES-III to insure a prespecified minimum sample size for each analytic domain so that estimates of the health and nutrition status of persons in each domain could be made with acceptable precision. The oversampling in NHANES-III was part of a pattern

3

established in the sample design. The population was decomposed into 52 subdomains: 7 age groups by sex for black and Mexican-American persons and 12 age groups by sex for white persons and other racial groups combined. After defining these age-sex-race/ethnicity subdomains, variable sampling rates were derived to ensure the achievement of sample sizes sufficient to permit analyses of the data for each subdomain."

NHANES is a valuable resource because it can support examination of public health issues that can best be addressed through physical examinations and laboratory tests. Each NHANES has a consistent core set of tests (e.g., height, weight, blood cholesterol) and questions (e.g., annual family income, race/ethnicity of subject) that are designed to assess the overall health and nutritional status of the subject and evaluate certain variables (e.g., socioeconomic status, SES) known to affect health and nutrition. Over the years, these core components have increased in number. During the planning phase of each NHANES, the collaborating agencies submit research proposals to NCHS requesting specific tests and/or questions to be administered to the subjects in addition to the core components. For example, in NHANES-III, EPA and the National Institute of Occupational Safety and Health (NIOSH) requested and had approval for lung function tests (e.g., spirometry) of subjects 8 years and older. Unlike the core components, agency-specific components will be retained in the survey only as long as there is mutual agreement between NCHS and the requesting funding agency to do so, and funding is available. Guidelines for preparing a proposal for submission to NCHS can be found on the following web site: <http://www.cdc.gov/nchs/data/prop02GL.pdf>. These guidelines were for proposals for the NHANES to be conducted in 2002, but are appropriate for future years of the survey.

All NHANES are cross-sectional surveys that use a complex, multistage, stratified design with cluster sampling to obtain a probability sample of people that is representative of the U.S. noninstitutionalized population. Although each NHANES provides a wealth of information on the prevalence of health conditions and risk factors, the cross-sectional nature of the original survey limits its usefulness for studying the effects of clinical, environmental, and behavioral variables on the development of specific health conditions. Data from follow-up surveys of original subjects are limited, but available, and can be used for examining health outcomes, primarily mortality (see Section 3.1). In addition, NHANES99+ data can be linked to Medicare and National Death Index records to permit longitudinal/historical studies of disease <http://www.cdc.gov/nchs/about/major/nhanes/current.htm>.

All NHANES are conducted in a similar manner. Subjects, called sample persons or SPs, are interviewed at home and this usually includes questions about the subject's personal health history; the family (i.e., income, ethnic heritage); and household characteristics (i.e., number of rooms in home, age of home). Subjects later go to a Mobile Examination Center (MEC) where standardized physical examinations are conducted by a doctor; blood is obtained by venipuncture of subjects ages 1 year and older and urine specimens are collected for individuals ages 6 years and older; and more questionnaires, including detailed questions about food preparation and consumption, are administered. There are now three MECs, each consisting of four large construction trailers, that travel around the country during the entire survey. At any point in time, only two MECs are set up and operating, while the third is either in transit or being set up. There are two teams of examiners responsible for staffing the MECs that are in operation in the field. Because of weather issues, the survey is generally conducted in northern areas during the summer and southern areas during the winter.

Each MEC is staffed with technicians, a doctor and a dentist and each is outfitted with computers, standardized laboratory facilities, examination rooms, and all the necessary equipment to conduct the various physiological tests. The clinical exams include evaluation of numerous analytes in the blood and urine, a medical examination by a doctor (including questions about past and current diseases and conditions), and other specialized tests (i.e., spirometry, computerized neurobehavioral testing). A limited number of tests are conducted on blood and urine samples at the MEC. Primarily blood and urine samples are processed at the MEC and then sent to specified labs for most of the analyses. The MECs stop at predetermined locations called "stands"(see Table 1). Each MEC stays at a particular stand for about 4-6 weeks during which time roughly 300- 600 subjects are evaluated. For more detailed information about the MEC and to take a virtual tour of the facility, go to the NCHS website at <http://www.cdc.gov/nchs/about/major/nhanes/mectour.htm#background>. Examples of the types of data collected in NHANES are as follows:

- demographics (e.g., age, sex, race/ethnicity, education, SES);
- housing and family characteristics (e.g., type/condition of house, number of occupants);
- risk factors (e.g., diet, physical activity, occupation, smoking habits);
- diseases of the subject and relatives (e.g., cardiovascular, respiratory, cancer, diabetes, kidney);
- reproductive history (e.g., number of children/pregnancies; age at onset of menses and menopause);
- detailed medical and dental examination;
- physiological tests (e.g., electrocardiogram (EKG), vision, hearing, neurobehavioral) ;
- anthropometric measurements (e.g., height, weight, girth, skin fold);
- clinical chemistries (assays of blood and urine, e.g., counts of various blood cell components, cholesterol level, levels of different vitamins in the blood, tests for kidney & liver function), see Appendices IV and VI for summaries of clinical chemistries for NHANES-III and NHANES99+, respectively. Also see Appendix V, for a comparison of clinical chemistries across NHANES-I, -II, -III and Hispanic HANES;
- environmental biochemistries (assays of blood and urine, e.g., blood lead levels, pesticides in urine, volatile organic compounds in blood, mercury in hair and blood.) Not all NHANES tested for the same chemicals, and the number of chemicals increased significantly in NHANES99+), see Appendix VII for comparison of environmental data collected across all NHANES;
- detailed nutrition questions (e.g., consumption of specific foods and dietary supplements, water intake, frequency of consuming specific foods), see Appendix IV for summary of dietary/nutritional evaluations from NHANES-III.

3.1. Followup Studies for the Baseline NHANES

NCHS has planned to conduct epidemiological follow-up studies (NHEFS) for each of the NHANES, but budget and staff limitations have severely curtailed these efforts. To date, NHEFS have only been conducted for NHANES-I (see Table 2). NHANES are cross-sectional studies that collect data on each subject at only one point in time. The objective of these followup studies is to obtain longitudinal data on all subjects that will support investigation of relationships among variables (e.g., demographic, clinical, nutritional, behavioral, and exposure) assessed in the original baseline NHANES and subsequent morbidity and mortality. For example, the data could be used to examine the association between certain risk factors (e.g., smoking, blood pressure, cholesterol, weight) and subsequent morbidity/mortality or to study the natural history of certain chronic diseases and functional impairment (e.g., why SPs with radiological evidence of osteoarthritis do, or do not, go on to develop functional impairment). Detailed information on the design, content, and operation of the NHEFS and access to the public use data files and documentation can be found on the following NCHS website: <http://www.cdc.gov/nchs/about/major/nhefs/nhefs.htm>.

In addition to the NHEFS, NCHS is also conducting the NHANES-II Mortality Study (NH2MS). This is a prospective cohort study designed to passively follow a subset of subjects from NHANES-II in order to investigate the association between factors measured at baseline and overall mortality from specific causes. The NH2MS mortality data can be linked with the baseline NHANES-II data to examine the relationship between any of the baseline variables (e.g., smoking, weight, blood lead, pesticides) and specific causes of death (NCHS, 1999a). The NH2MS cohort contains adults who were 30-75 years of age at the time of their NHANES-II examination (N=9,252). During the baseline NHANES-II, some participants were interviewed but not examined; however, only those examined at baseline were followed for mortality status. During this first Phase of the study, mortality status was ascertained for years 1976-92. The NH2MS cohort members were traced by searching national databases containing mortality and cause-of-death information. The length of followup period ranges from 12 to 16 years. Approximately 23 percent (n=2,145) of the NH2MS cohort were found to be deceased as of December 31, 1992.

The design of NH2MS differs substantially from that of the NHEFS, since the latter was an active followup study with participants being recontacted and medical records and death certificates being obtained. In contrast, the NH2MS is entirely passive, with participants not being recontacted and not all death certificates being obtained. Mortality status in NH2MS was ascertained solely by computerized matching to national databases and evaluation of the resulting matches. Matching to the National Death Index (NDI) and other national databases will continue on a periodic basis, with resulting data being released to the public. One important limitation of the NH2MS design is that subjects not found to be deceased are assumed alive for analytic purposes, and this could cause a misclassification of vital status.

Detailed information on the design, content, and operation of the 1992 NH2MS is in the Vital and Health Statistics Series 1, Number 38 "Plan and Operation of the NHANES II Mortality Study 1992"(NCHS, 1999a). This document, plus the public use data file and

6

documentation can be found at the NCHS website: <http://www.cdc.gov/nchs/products/catalogs/subject/nh2ms.htm>.

3.2. How NHANES have been used to Improve Public Health

NHANES have provided much valuable data that have been used over the years to improve public health. Some examples noted on the NCHS website <http://www.cdc.gov/nchs/about/major/nhanes/DataAccomp.htm> are as follows: a) development of growth charts that are used nationally and internationally by physicians as standards for assessing the growth of their young patients; b) assessment by the U.S. Department of Agriculture (USDA) of the vitamin and mineral intake of the population and use of this information to improve our diets. Earlier NHANES showed that low iron levels were a serious problem for many people, including women of childbearing age, preschool children, and the elderly. As a result, the government took steps to fortify grain and cereal with iron to correct this deficiency; c) NHANES showed the need for folate to eliminate another dietary deficiency and prevent birth defects; d) For years, NHANES has tracked the levels of cholesterol in adults. This information has helped to establish the link between high cholesterol levels and the risk of heart disease and to alert patients and doctors to the issue. When NHANES started testing, one-third of adults had high cholesterol, but today fewer than 1 in 5 adults do. Changes in diet and lifestyle all built on information from the national survey have sharply reduced the risk of dying from a heart attack; e) NHANES-II (1976-80) gave the first clear-cut evidence of the high levels of blood lead (PbB) in the U.S. population, particularly in children. This evidence led congress, the EPA, and other agencies to phase out the use of lead (Pb) as an additive in gasoline and the resulting reduction in PbB levels has been remarkable. These data were also used to support federal policies to eliminate Pb from solder in food and soft drink cans. Monitoring of PbB levels in NHANES-III and NHANES99+ show a continued decrease in the body burdens of this toxicant. Pb exposure remains a problem for certain groups, especially poor, inner city children living in old houses with lead paint. NHANES99+ continues to monitor for PbB and this information helps public health agencies pinpoint where Pb remains a problem; f) NHANES data continue to indicate that undiagnosed diabetes is a significant problem in the U.S.. The data have been used by federal and private agencies to increase public awareness, especially among minorities, of this problem; and g) NHANES has produced information on the prevalence of overweight and obesity that have led to the proliferation of programs emphasizing diet and exercise and stimulated needed research. New measures of physical fitness used in NHANES99+ will further our understanding of its role in health and enhance the analysis of relationships among exercise, obesity and disease. For more information on how NHANES has been, and will be used to improve public health, see the above-noted website. Also, see Section 6.2 of this Handbook for more information on how NHANES has been used to support risk assessment, policy needs and regulatory decisions at EPA.

4.0. DETAILED INFORMATION ON NHANES CONTENT

NHANES is the largest survey for gathering data on the health and nutritional status of the U.S. population. It is designed to facilitate and encourage subject participation, by providing transportation to and from the MEC and compensating subjects for their time and effort. Each participant also receives a report of their medical and dental findings. In addition, NCHS goes to great lengths to study the reasons why potential subjects do, or do not, participate in the survey. The information obtained is used to devise tactics for increasing response rates (e.g., increased local media coverage; increased targeting of specific race/ethnicity groups with appropriately tailored publicity). These efforts have paid off, as indicated by the steadily increasing response rates with each successive survey. Thus, the overall response rates (including interview and MEC examination) have increased as follows: NHANES-II (73.1%), HHANES (73.3%), NHANES-III (76.6%) and NHANES99+ (78%) (Source: NHANES Consortium meeting, 2002).

As noted in Section 3.0, all data are gathered through personal interviews, physical examinations, and diagnostic and biochemical testing of a statistically representative sample of the U.S. population. Also as noted in Section 3.0, there is a core set of components that is administered in each of the NHANES and there are agency-specific components that are retained as long as there is mutual interest between NCHS and the requesting agency to do so, and funding is available. Over the years, the number of tests and questions administered to subjects has greatly increased. Of the completed surveys (NHANES-I, -II, -III and HHANES), NHANES-III is the most recent and collected the largest amount of data. Although the field work for NHANES-99 and -01 has been finished, analysis of blood and urine samples has not been completed for many analytes, and data have not been released to the public (see Section 4.0 and Table 3 for data release schedule for NHANES-99 - 08). For these reasons, this Handbook presents detailed examples of the survey content from NHANES-III and then presents summary information comparing specific components across the surveys. By becoming familiar with the details of NHANES-III, the reader will have a sound understanding of the basic characteristics of all the NHANES.

Appendix II provides an overview of the health status assessment component of NHANES-III by describing the public health objectives and data collected to support the following: 1) evaluation of the health of specific population subgroups, such as children and adolescents, the elderly, women and minorities; 2) assessment of environmental and occupational health and exposures; 3) evaluation of specific diseases (e.g., cardiovascular, respiratory, diabetes); and 4) examination of specific risk factors (e.g., smoking, alcohol and tobacco use). More information on the design and data collection of NHANES-III and public use data files can be found on the NCHS website: <http://www.cdc.gov/nchs/about/major/nhanes/datalink.htm>. This website also contains links to comparable information for all the surveys. Just click on the name of the specific survey for access to manuals, documentation books and data files.

Appendix III provides an overview of the nutritional status assessment component of NHANES-III by describing the data collected to support the following: 1) evaluation of alcohol intake; 2) assessment of hunger; 3) examination of vitamin and mineral status through biochemical testing of blood and urine; 4) evaluation of infant and child nutrition; 5) evaluation of growth, overweight and obesity; and 6) examination of relationships between diet and health. Appendix III also summarizes the methods employed for obtaining the nutritional data, including questions about food frequency and the 24-hour dietary recall; measures of anthropometry; and laboratory determinations. More information on the design and data collection of the nutritional component of NHANES-III and public use data files can be found at <http://www.cdc.gov/nchs/about/major/nhanes/datalink.htm>. As noted above, this website contains links to comparable information for all the surveys.

Appendix IV summarizes the tests and questions administered in NHANES-III. This Appendix includes a description, by age of subject, of the following: 1) questionnaire topics; 2) physical examination components; 3) analytes tested in blood and urine; 4) special studies, including a list of volatile organic compounds (VOCs) tested in the blood of a random sample of adults; and 5) dietary and nutrition intake information.

Given the complexity of the NHANES, it is difficult to summarize information about the entire content of individual surveys in order to compare components across all surveys. Appendix V compares the clinical chemistries in blood and urine for NHANES-I, -II, -III and HHANES. Appendix VI compares only the components of the current survey for the years 1999-2002, as follows: Table 1 compares the analyses in blood, urine and hair, by year and subject age; Table 2 compares questionnaire content by year and subject age; Table 3 compares examination components by year and subject age.

As indicated in Sections 3.0 and 4.0, each NHANES has collected a certain amount of environmental and risk factor data that have potential interest to EPA. With each successive survey, collection of these types of data has increased markedly. Appendix VII presents a comparison of environmentally relevant data collected across all the NHANES, by age of subjects. This includes questions asked about potential exposures (e.g., smoking history, use of pesticides in garden and home) and identification of specific biomarkers in blood, urine, hair and environmental media. With increasing concerns about environmental exposures and the possible link between exposures and health effects and/or decrements in physiological functioning, there is increasing interest in collecting needed exposure data through NHANES. Now, and into the future, NHANES99+ will be collecting a tremendous amount of environmental biomarker data that have potential interest to EPA. Because of the expense of the various tests and the finite amount of bodily fluids that can be obtained from each subject, it is not possible to conduct all analyses on every subject, so only subsamples may be tested. For all chemicals, the size of subsamples is noted , such as "1/3 sample", which means that 1/3 of the age-eligible subjects were tested. Analysis of many of the analytes listed in Appendix VII for NHANES99+ will continue through at least 2002. Check the NCHS website <http://www.cdc.gov/nchs /nhanes.htm> for updates on specific chemicals to be evaluated in the future years.

Data from NHANES99+ have not yet been released to the public or collaborating agencies, and none are expected for release until later in 2002. However, NCHS and CDC have conducted some preliminary analyses on the limited data, primarily from NHANES-99. Reports summarizing these limited analyses can be found on the following NCHS website: <http://www.cdc.gov/nchs/about/major/nhanes/findings.htm>. Currently, the listed reports include: *Blood and Hair Mercury Levels in Young Children and Women of Childbearing Age-- U.S. 1999; Blood Lead Levels in Young Children– United States and Selected States–1996-1999;*

Folate Status in Women of Childbearing Age-- United States, 1999; Prevalence of Overweight Among Children and Adolescents– United States, 1999; and Prevalence of Overweight and Obesity Among Adults– United States, 1999. This website also contains the *National Report on Human Exposure to Environmental Chemicals*, a new CDC publication started in March, 2001and described as providing an ongoing assessment of the U.S. population's exposure to environmental chemicals using biomonitoring. This *Report* uses NHANES99+ blood and urine biomonitoring data to provide statistical summaries of levels of environmental chemicals in the people. Depending on the amount of raw data, these summaries may, or may not, be categorized by age, race, SES, or other characteristics of the population. CDC plans to release this *Report* every year based on new NHANES data. For some EPA offices these statistical summaries may be sufficient to support regulatory and/or policy needs.

5.0 HOW TO OBTAIN NHANES DATA AND ISSUES WITH FILE STRUCTURE AND CONTENT

NCHS works with the collaborating agencies to QA/QC the field data and then generates files for all the clinical, laboratory and questionnaire data for each subject. NCHS generates various weighting factors and other documentation needed to analyze the data and develops data sets that are periodically released to the collaborating agencies and then to the public. NCHS does not release any confidential subject information that could be used to identify the subject or his/her residential location. All of the publicly available data from all the NHANES, including the NHEFS and the 1992 HANES-II Mortality Study, can now be obtained either over the Internet, through the NCHS Research Data Center (See Section 5.2) or ordered from the National Technical Information Service (NTIS). The NCHS website <http://www.cdc.gov/nchs/about /major/nhanes/datalink.htm> provides links for obtaining the data and documentation on-line and instructions for ordering materials from NTIS. Just click on the name of the specific survey for access to manuals, documentation books and data files.

NCHS also provides survey-specific reports, manuals and other documentation that are needed to understand the survey design, methodological issues, components of the survey and how the different components were conducted. These documents are available for all the NHANES through <http://www.cdc.gov/nchs/about/major/nhanes/datalink.htm>, or from NTIS, and include the following:

> 1) <u>Plan and Operation Books</u> contain a detailed overview of the specific survey and provide descriptive information on specific components of the health status and nutritional assessments; sample design and analysis guidelines; data collection procedures; a copy of the interview forms; and a list of exam components.

> 2) <u>Documentation Books</u> are provided with the data files. They contain a list of the exam/interview components that are in each data file; guidance on how to use the data files; information on how to create datasets from the data files; data preparation and processing procedures; descriptions of the variable names used and positional location of

each variable in the data files; and raw counts of subjects for each survey question, lab component and test.

   3) <u>Interviewer Procedure Manuals</u> were developed for training the interviewers and are important references for NHANES as they detail the correct procedures, policies, and standards for interacting with the subjects while conducting the interviews.

   4) <u>Exam Manuals</u> detail the correct procedures and equipment used for administering each physiological test and the questionnaires.

   Now that NHANES is an annual survey that will be in the field continuously, NCHS has had to deal with many new issues regarding frequency of data release. For example, since only 5,000 subjects are examined each year, there are questions about the number of subjects needed to calculate statistically meaningful estimates from the data. With this small number of annual subjects, there are also issues about protection of subject confidentiality. At the 2002 Consortium meeting of the federal agencies supporting NHANES, NCHS announced new plans for scheduling not only raw data releases, but survey planning activities and report releases (see Table 3). From now on, all these activities will be conducted on a 2-year cycle (1999-2000, 2001-2002, 2003-2004, etc.). "Micro-data", identified as all the raw sociodemographic, exam, and questionnaire data, will not be released for single years of the survey because of concerns about protecting subject confidentiality. "Tabular Reports" will be prepared by NCHS and/or CDC to summarize findings on a limited number of variables judged to be of significant public health importance. These Tabular Reports, unlike the raw data, will be based one year's worth of data and will be released annually. NCHS will now solicit proposals for new survey components, and pilot test certain proposed components, on this 2-year cycle. Many data elements (e.g., residential location, data collected on a small subset of subjects) will never be made available to the public in order to protect subject confidentiality. These data are often very valuable and critical to support studies of public, and/or environmental health importance, and studies that can support EPA regulatory, policy and/or research needs. As indicated in Table 3, NCHS is scheduled to make these data available only through their Research Data Center (RDC). See Section 5.2 of this Handbook for details on the RDC and how to access the data.

5.1. Issues with Data File Structure and Content
   Each NHANES provides an incredibly rich source of human data for research and analysis. However, the data set is large, complex and requires that the user be familiar with data file manipulation and analysis. Thorough review of the extensive documentation provided by NCHS for the individual datasets should resolve most questions. All data users need to review these reference materials and reports before analyzing any NHANES data. If you still have questions after careful review of the documentation, try contacting the NCHS Data Dissemination Branch at (301)458-4636.

   The following examples demonstrate the complexity of the data file structure and content and illustrate some of the many issues that need to be considered when designing a study using data from any NHANES:

11

●Data from each NHANES are divided into separate files. Depending on the analysis to be performed, one or more of these files will need to be merged in order to obtain all the needed data on each subject. Users need to be familiar with the content of each file. For example, the NHANES-III survey design and demographic variables are in the Household Adult Data File (subjects 18+ years old), Household Youth Data File (subjects up to 17 years old), Laboratory Data File (all ages), and Examination Data File (all ages). All of the NHANES-III public use data files are linked through the common survey participant identification number (sample sequence number or SEQN). Merging information from multiple NHANES-III data files using the SEQN variable ensures that the appropriate information for each subject is linked correctly. In preparing a data set for analysis, other data files should be merged with the Adult Household Data File and/or the Youth Household Data File to obtain many important analytic variables.

● NHANES public use data files do not have the same number of records on each file. For example, in NHANES-III the Adult and Youth Household Questionnaire Files contain more records than the Examination Data File because not everyone who was interviewed went on to complete the examination. The Laboratory Data File contains data only for persons aged one year and older. The Individual Foods Data File based on the dietary recall, the Prescription Medication Data File, and the Vitamin and Minerals Data File, all have multiple records for each person rather than the one record per subject contained in the other data files.

● With each data file, NCHS includes separate text files with SAS program code using standard variable names and labels. This SAS program code can be used to create SAS data sets from the data file.

● During the course of each NHANES, NCHS modifies items in the questionnaires, laboratory, and/or examination components. As a result, data may not be available for certain variables for all years of any one survey. In addition, variables may differ by the phase of the survey because some changes were implemented between phases. For example, NHANES-III was conducted in two phases from 1988-1991 and 1991-1994. Because of the changing research needs of the sponsoring agencies, NCHS dropped a limited number of questions and examination components after the first phase, and replaced these with new questions and tests in the second phase. This process of survey modification will become more noticeable with NHANES99+, since the survey is now in the field continuously, and proposals for new components will be on a two year cycle (see Table 3). In general, if new components are added, then old component(s) need to be deleted so the burden to subjects is not significantly increased. Furthermore, NCHS is currently trying to determine how many years specific components should be retained in order to obtain a statistically meaningful sample size. Because of these modifications, users need to read the Notes sections of the file documentation carefully, as they provide information about survey changes.

● NCHS verifies extremely high and low test values whenever possible, and performs numerous consistency checks on the data. Nonetheless, users need to examine the range and frequency of values before analyzing data.

● Confidential and administrative data are not available or released to the public. (See Section 5.2 on how these data may be accessed through the NCHS Data Research Center). Additionally, some variables have been recoded to protect the confidentiality of the survey participants. For example, in NHANES-III all age-related variables were recoded to 90+ years for persons who were 90 years of age or older.

See the following website for more information on guidelines for NHANES data users based on NHANES-III: <ftp://ftp.cdc.gov/pub/Health_Statistics/NCHS/Datasets/NHANES/NHANESIII /11A/readme.txt>.

5.2. NCHS Research Data Center (RDC)

As already noted, there is no public release of any confidential data on NHANES subjects; however, NCHS collects and maintains these data (such as residential address). Without access to certain types of confidential information, it would be impossible to conduct some types of studies that would be very useful to EPA. For example, if one just uses the publicly available data, analyses are generally limited to a national or regional scale, or to comparisons made for urban vs rural areas. It should be noted that while the design and release of NHANES data limit analyses to these large geographic scales, in many cases this is sufficient and appropriate for EPA needs. A case in point was EPA's use of NHANES-II data to develop the distribution of blood lead (PbB) levels in children for the whole country in support of regulations to reduce Pb in gasoline (U.S.DHH, 1988; U.S. EPA, 1986).

NCHS recently established a Research Data Center (RDC) at its headquarters in Hyattsville, Maryland. More detailed information about the RDC, its rules for prospective users, and how to access it can be found at <http://www.cdc.gov/nchs/r&d/rdc.htm>. Briefly, the RDC was created to meet the continuing demand for analyses to be conducted on smaller geographical scales (e.g., by state, county and below county) that require restricted data from NHANES. Designed for the researcher outside of NCHS, the RDC allows access to data that would not be permissible to analyze because of confidentiality/disclosure rules and regulations. These sensitive data can not be publicly released, but potentially can be accessed through the RDC, for statistical studies. In addition, the potential exists for linking NHANES data to environmental data, as noted above, but also to other human databases, such as the Census data and the National Death Index. By working through the RDC, it will be possible to link NHANES data to a variety of other data bases in order to expand the usefulness of NHANES and conduct studies not possible if just based on NHANES data alone. Data sets for linking can be user-generated (e.g., exposure data generated from environmental monitors), or publicly available (e.g., Census data). Only the RDC staff can link the data sets. Files and information used to link any data sets are destroyed after the merged file is created and are not be made available to the user.

The RDC has instituted restricted conditions to protect sensitive data but allow analyses at a level not possible with public use data. These conditions are identified on the website

<http://www.cdc.gov/nchs/r&d/rdc.htm> and summarized as follows:

1) Prospective researchers must submit a research proposal to the RDC for review and approval. Approval will be based on the availability of RDC staff and resources; consistency of the proposal with the mission of NCHS; general scientific soundness of the proposal; and the feasibility of the project. It is expected that the user will develop the research proposal with the RDC staff to minimize the time required.

2) Researchers will sign confidentiality agreements, but strict confidentiality protocols require that researchers with approved projects must complete their work using the RDC facilities. RDC facilities can be accessed on-site or remotely.

3) Researchers can supply their own data to be merged by RDC staff with NCHS data sets. Merged files will be only available to the originating researcher unless written permission is given to allow access to others.

The RDC can be accessed on-site, in Hyattsville, MD or remotely. Another analysis option for researchers with large, complex analytic projects may be to subcontract with the RDC to have its staff run the necessary programs, etc. for the research project. Each mode of access has associated costs, procedures, rules and limitations. Other details of the RDC operation are discussed on the website <http://www.cdc.gov/nchs/r&d/rdc.htm> as follows:

For on-site users:
● RDC staff will construct necessary data files, including those linking NHANES data with user data.
● PC SAS, SUDAAN, STATA, FORTRAN and HLM are available. Other statistical packages are available with sufficient lead time for RDC staff.
● Output is subject to disclosure review by the RDC staff. Disclosure review guidelines are published in the NCHS Staff Manual on Confidentiality.
● Analyses (paper output) can be taken off site contingent on passing disclosure review by RDC staff.
● The RDC is only open during normal working hours and requires RDC staff oversight.

For remote access users:
● RDC staff will construct necessary data files, including those linking NHANES data with user data.
● Researchers can submit analytical computer programs via e-mail. Output is returned by e-mail to users' registered address.
● Only SAS programs can be run. Certain SAS procedures and functions are not allowed, including: PROC TABULATE, PROC IML, LIST and PRINT (e.g., no listing of individual cases), R_, FIRST., LAST., (e.g., no selection of individual cases). No cell with fewer than five observations can be included; and if found, other cells will also be suppressed.
● The SAS job log will be scanned for conditions that result in case listings.

Specific costs:
- To work on site costs a researcher $1,000 per week.
- To remotely access any one data set costs $500 per month.
- File construction and setup by RDC staff for either remote access or on-site use costs $500 per day of effort.

6.0.   TYPES OF ANALYSES THAT CAN BE CONDUCTED WITH NHANES DATA

NHANES can be a valuable resource for EPA to use in support of research, risk assessment, policy decisions and regulations. This rich human database has several features that make it attractive for EPA use, including: 1) potential to be linked with other databases, including census, exposure and mortality data; 2) can be used to identify emerging health and exposure issues; 3) can be used to examine associations between possible risk factors and adverse health effects or other conditions; 4) can be used to help evaluate the effectiveness of existing environmental regulations and the need for additional/new regulations; 5) can be used to investigate issues based on race/ethnicity and SES (e.g., environmental equity issues) and geographic location; and 6) potential for limited longitudinal studies as more follow-up data are collected (see Section 3.1).

Different methods can be used examine the NHANES data, including the following:

1) Development of population distributions of specific variables (e.g., height, weight, PbB, blood or urine levels of environmental chemicals). These distributions can be developed for the U.S. population as a whole, or for specific subgroups based on a variety of characteristics such as age, race/ethnicity, SES, gender, etc. It should also be possible to develop distributions for different parts of the country, but this may need to be accomplished through the Research Data Center (see Section 5.2).

2) Estimation of the prevalence of selected diseases or chronic conditions (e.g., respiratory, cardiovascular, neurobehavioral). Prevalences can be calculated for the U.S. population as a whole, or for various subgroups. Subgroups can be defined by demographic characteristics, or with assistance from the RDC using characteristics of their residential neighborhoods (see Section 5.2).

3) Use of inferential studies to examines possible associations between various risk factors and particular diseases or conditions. For example, based on NHANES-III data, one can assess potential risk factors (e.g., active and passive smoking, allergies to cats/dogs, use of gas stove) for asthma in children, and assess the value of these risk factors as predictors for asthma.

Because of the design of NHANES, there are limitations on how estimates can be expressed. For example, analyses can be developed based on:

1) National estimates (e.g., distribution of PbB levels for all children 1-5 years of age).

2) Estimates by broad geographic regions (NE, NW, SE, etc.), (e.g., distribution of PbB levels for all children 1-5 years of age and living in the south).

3) Estimates by degree of urbanization (e.g., distribution of PbB levels for children 1-5 years of age living in metropolitan areas vs rural areas).

4) Estimates by other major population subgroups, such as race/ethnicity, income, sex, or age (e.g., distribution of PbB levels in black children ages 1-5 years compared to Hispanic children of the same age).

With the advent of geographic information systems (GIS), it is now possible to geographically locate point and area sources of pollution; map plumes of pollutants in the air, groundwater and soil; and model and map other environmental exposures. It should also be possible to link NHANES data, through appropriate geographical identifiers, with mapped environmental data in order to evaluate possible relationships between variables in the human data and exposures from the environmental data. For example, NCEA is collaborating with NCHS to conduct a study of risk factors for respiratory effects in children by linking EPA air monitoring data with NHANES-III children's respiratory data. The addresses of the children have been geocoded to the Census block group level by NCHS and the monitoring data for ozone and PM10 have been interpolated to the block group level by NCEA. NCHS links both sets of data by the common field of census block group and then retains the linked data set to protect subject confidentiality. The linked data are used to evaluate relationships between exposure to these air pollutants and respiratory effects, including decrements in lung function (See APPENDIX IX, project summary entitled "Estimation of Risk Factors for Respiratory Effects in Children: Use of NHANES-III Respiratory Health and EPA Air Monitoring Data. Part IV). The block group identification of the NHANES-III subjects is confidential and not released to the public, but is part of the data set. Any publications resulting from this study will not disclose the locations of the NHANES children. Moreover, it is important to note that given the design of NHANES-III (and all NHANES), the results of this study can only be expressed as whether or not ozone and/or PM10 have an effect on the respiratory health of children. The design of NHANES will not support an analysis of whether children in specific parts (i.e., cities, counties, states) of the country have poorer lung function because they live in an area with "high" air pollution levels. The design of NHANES will support an analysis to determine if, in general, higher levels of air pollution are associated with poorer respiratory health in children. Provided that subject confidentiality is maintained and the type of analysis is consistent with the design of NHANES, the possibility exists for conducting similar types of studies by linking NHANES data to other environmental databases. See Section 8.0 for more precautions on appropriate use of NHANES data. Now that the NCHS RDC (See Section 5.2) has been established, it should be possible, with the appropriate data, to conduct these types of studies.

6.1. Studies using NHANES Data that have Environmental Relevance

Many papers have been published using NHANES data and these cover a wide variety of topics, many of which are of potential interest to EPA. NCHS maintains an annotated bibliography of the studies they are aware of; however, this list is not exhaustive. Annual updates to this bibliography and copies of NCHS/CDC publications cited in the bibliography may be obtained from the Data Dissemination Branch, NCHS, 6525 Belcrest Road, Hyattsville, Maryland 20782. A selective bibliography from 1997 -1999 can be found on the following NCHS website: <http://www.cdc.gov/nchs/about/major/nhanes/97-99jan00.pdf>.

Based on the bibliography from the NCHS website, plus another selective bibliography NCHS prepared for 1980-1996 but that is not on their website, we have assembled a list of references (See APPENDIX VIII) that have potential environmental relevance. Note that Appendix VIII contains a mix of annotated references, which were taken from the NCHS 1997-1999 bibliography and references without annotation, which were taken from the NCHS 1980-1996 bibliography. This compilation of references also provides a good overview of the broad range of studies that can be conducted with NHANES data.

6.2. Use of NHANES Data at EPA

Over the years, EPA has successfully used NHANES data in research and to support policy and regulatory decisions. Some of these activities included:

1) Evaluation of the relationship between PbB, adverse health effects (e.g., cognitive function, hypertension) and levels of Pb in the environment, particularly as a result of Pb in gasoline. NHANES-II data were used to support EPA regulations to remove Pb from gasoline. NHANES data also demonstrated decreases in PbB that paralleled decreases in Pb in gasoline. EPA monitors Pb exposures by evaluating NHANES-III and NHANES99+ PbB data and uses these data to support continuing policy decisions. (U.S.DHHS, 1988; U.S.EPA, 1986). Also see Appendix IX.

2) Evaluation of respiratory function and persistent respiratory symptom data from NHANES-I and -II. EPA used these data to support regulatory decisions for the National Ambient Air Quality Standards (NAAQS) pollutants, which include ozone, sulfur oxides, nitrogen oxides, particulate matter, lead and carbon monoxide.

3) Evaluation of NHANES99+ data on mercury (Hg) levels in blood and hair of children and women of child-bearing age. These data are used by several EPA offices to determine exposure levels to methyl-mercury in these two susceptible subpopulations and to support policy decisions on Hg exposures. EPA will continue to use these data to support policy and regulatory decisions, as the levels for subjects tested in 2000 and beyond are made publicly available (See Appendix IX).

4) Use of HHANES urine and serum pesticide data to develop distributions of the prevalence of pesticide exposures in Hispanic subpopulations. These distributions were used as reference standards for assessing pesticide exposures in children and adults in studies of populations living along the U.S.- Mexico border.

5) Use of urine and serum pesticide data in combination with food consumption data to support development of pesticide tolerance levels in food.

17

6) Evaluation of pulmonary function for different population subgroups based on age, sex, and race. EPA used these data to develop predictive models for several spirometric endpoints (e.g., FEV_1, FVC) for children, teens, and young adults. The models allow for investigation of how pulmonary function differs by race and sex and how these differences interact with growth and development patterns.

7) Examination of the relationship between blood pressure and the level of cadmium (Cd) in urine, which is an indicator of the body burden of Cd. Work has also included examining the correlation between Cd in urine and beta2-microglobulin (indicator of Cd-induced renal damage) and using the information as benchmarks for measuring the effects of environmental Cd exposure.

8) Use of surplus blood sera from NHANES-III subjects to determine if poorer drinking water quality correlated with higher prevalence of antibodies to *Cryptosporidium* (see Appendix IX).

Several EPA program offices currently use NHANES data in epidemiology studies and/or to support policy and regulatory work. APPENDIX IX presents summaries of twenty two EPA efforts we were aware of that use NHANES data. Again, note the broad diversity of issues being addressed and different methods being applied to the data.

7.0. USE OF NHANES STORED BIOLOGICAL SPECIMENS

7.1. Serum Specimens:
Blood collected from NHANES-III subjects was separated into its components and sent to the CDC laboratory or to one of the eight contract laboratories for testing (see Appendices IV and VII). Because of the possibility of out-of-range results that need to be repeated, more specimen volume was sent to the labs than was usually needed for the scheduled biochemical tests. Since most subjects do not have out-of-range results, the labs now have a large numbers of surplus serum specimens. All specimens have been stored at -70 degrees and have been through at least two freeze-thaw cycles. Stored sera from NHANES-III are available for research projects that require a nationally representative sample of the population. Research proposals are accepted and reviewed throughout the year by the NHANES-III Stored Sera Technical Review Panel, which attempts to review the proposals within 30 days of receipt. See the NCHS website <http://www.cdc.gov/nchs/about/major/nhanes/serum1a.htm> for more details on the proposal solicitation process; review process; proposal selection criteria; and guidelines for proposal preparation.

Note that EPA has successfully used NHANES-III serum samples to conduct a study of the relationship between serum antibody response to *Cryptosporidium* and the primary source and treatment of drinking water. See Appendix IX, study entitled "Analysis of Serological Responses to *Cryptosporidium* Antigen Among NHANES-III Participants" for a summary of this work.

In NHANES99+, samples of blood, urine, and saliva (if applicable) for subjects 7 years and older who give their written consent are being stored for future health studies <http://www.cdc.gov/nchs/about/major/nhanes/00futstu.pdf>.

7.2. DNA Samples:

For NHANES-III subjects 12 years of age and older, lymphocytes (white cells) were isolated from blood samples and stored frozen in liquid nitrogen or as cell cultures immortalized with Epstein-Barr virus. The cells have been stored and maintained at the Division of Environmental Health Laboratory Sciences (DEHLS) at the National Center for Environmental Health (NCEH), CDC. Cell cultures are available primarily from Phase 2 of the survey, which was conducted 1991-1994. Though an extensive consent form was signed by participants in the survey, specific mention of genetic testing was not included. Collection and storage of this biological material was based on the promise offered by significant advances in the rapidly evolving field of molecular biology that were occurring during the NHANES-III planning phase. Technical advances now make it possible to use these specimens for genetic analysis. NCHS and NCEH are making anonymized DNA from these specimens available to the research community for such analyses, but no cell lines will be made available.

Given the scientific importance of this resource, NCHS developed a plan for making DNA samples available to the research community for anonymized testing. This plan was approved by the NHANES Institutional Review Board (IRB) September 16, 1996. For more details and guidelines concerning development, submission, review and acceptance of proposals for studies using stored DNA samples, see the following NCHS web site: <http://www.cdc.gov/nchs/about/major/nhanes/dnafnlgm2.htm>. This website now indicates that since the Fall of 2001, NCHS is in the process of reevaluating their protocol for soliciting and approving proposals for studies using the stored DNA specimens. The website further indicates that their ultimate goal is to allow reasonable access to the samples for important scientific studies while assuring participant confidentiality and compliance with appropriate ethical standards. For these reasons, NCHS has discontinued further review of applications while they revise their protocol. If the revised protocol is approved by the NHANES IRB, they will place an announcement on the above-noted web site, and presumably start accepting proposals again.

In NHANES99+, DNA samples (from blood or saliva) from subjects ages 20 and over who give their written consent are being stored for future genetic testing <http://www.cdc.gov/nchs/about/major/nhanes/00futstu.pdf>.

8.0. LIMITATIONS AND PRECAUTIONS ON USE OF NHANES DATA

The analysis of NHANES data is not a straightforward task. "The analyst must consider many issues to develop an appropriate and efficient strategy for conducting the analysis. Such considerations should include ...the sample design, weights, or underlying assumptions in the analytic procedures to be applied..." (NCHS, 1982). Before starting any analysis using NHANES data, researchers need to be aware of several key issues:

A) Goals of NHANES vs goals of studies analyzing NHANES data— a geographical perspective.

Although there are many important issues to be considered when designing a study using NHANES data, one of the most critical deals with the incorporation of geographical information and the appropriateness of using NHANES data to examine health effects and risk factors on a small scale. Remember that the goal of NHANES is to provide information on the health and nutritional status of the U.S. population. The complex design of NHANES has been developed to support that goal. Because this is a unique survey that provides such a wealth of data on such a large number of people, it is easy to overlook this goal and try to conduct analyses that are of interest to EPA but may be inappropriate given the design of NHANES. A prime example of this potential pitfall is based on the fact that NHANES is conducted in numerous locations (e.g., stands), with several hundred people examined at each location (See Section 3.0 and Table 1). NCHS also publicly identifies the county of residence, provided the population is greater than 500,000. Because of this geographical distribution of subjects, you may be tempted to identify stands that are located "near" hazardous waste sites or specific industrial point sources of pollution that are of interest to EPA and then conduct an analysis to see if there is a correlation between adverse health effects and living "near" a particular pollution source. NHANES was not designed to support this type of study, because the people examined at a particular stand are not necessarily representative of the population in that immediate area. Although we now have techniques (e.g., GIS) that allow for creative ways to incorporate geographic detail into analyses of NHANES data, these approaches may not always be valid, given the design and underlying purpose of this survey. With GIS it is now possible to access many environmentally-relevant databases (e.g., locations of point and area sources of pollution) or generate your own (e.g., model air concentrations of chemicals released from a specific industry or industries) and then link these to the NHANES data in order to explore hypotheses about risk factors for adverse health effects at specific locations. While many such interesting analyses are possible, are they always appropriate? Remember, NHANES is designed to support estimates of effects, etc. based on: a) a national level; b) a broad regional level (e.g., NE, NW, SE); c) by degree of urbanization (e.g., metropolitan areas vs rural settings); d) by population subgroup (e.g., race/ethnicity, income, sex, age). NHANES is not designed to provide valid parameter estimates based on survey participants living in specific locations such as local towns, counties or states. NHANES was not designed to support studies of the health status of individuals in a specific location. Thus, when developing a study that uses NHANES data, you need to ensure that the design of your study is consistent with the goals and design of NHANES and makes appropriate use of the data (NCHS, 1982; and the following website: <http://www.cdc.gov/nceh/dls/report/totalreport/datasources.htm>.

B) Complex sample design of NHANES.

NHANES uses a complex, stratified, multistage, probability cluster design to select a representative sample of the noninstitutionalized, civilian U.S. population. Because of this complicated design, one can not use traditional statistical methods to analyze the data

C) Need for weighting.

Because the NHANES sample design is complex, sample weights must be used to account for stratification, clustering, and the unequal probability of subject selection into the survey. Each NHANES oversamples certain population subgroups (see Section 3.0 and Table1), and this must be taken into account through appropriate weighting. Sample weights are also used to adjust for possible bias resulting from subject nonresponse. Weighting is used to bring the sample data up to the dimensions of the target population totals and to reduce variances in estimations. The issue of using weights is critical to the correct analysis of NHANES data. NCHS calculates the necessary weights for different components of the survey and provides these with the public use datasets, along with explanations of how the weights were derived and when to use them. It is the responsibility of the user to select the appropriate weights and apply them correctly. There is also an issues of whether or not to use certain weights, depending on the type of analysis being conducted. Inappropriate use of weights may result in a flawed analysis and questionable study results. See Section 9.1 for more information about weighting.

D) Limitations associated with small sample size.

As noted elsewhere (see issue E, "Variable content within surveys", of Section 8.0 and Appendices VI and VII) some variables are measured only in subsamples of the survey and/or for a limited time. Moreover, because each NHANES is conducted over multiple years, it may be enticing to try to examine time trends by making and comparing annual estimates within a particular survey. Any of these conditions may result in having a small sample size for one or more variables and this complicates analysis of the data and interpretation of the results. This problem of small sample size is illustrated by the CDC's analysis of the first year of the NHANES99+ biomonitoring data for their *National Report on Human Exposure to Environmental Chemicals* (see Section 4.0 and the following website: <http://www.cdc.gov/nceh/dls/report/totalreport /datasources.htm>). This *Report* indicates:

> "Although the current NHANES is conducted using annual samples that are nationally representative, the sample size in any one year is relatively small, resulting in large variability for estimates, especially those for detailed demographic groups or other detailed analyses. The NHANES is designed to increase precision by combining data across calendar years. Because of the small sample size in 1999, a number of survey participants have large sample weights, and the potential exists that these sample weights may strongly influence estimates. This is particularly important for chemical results that were only measured in subsamples."

> "Another analytic limitation of the NHANES sample is that it is selected from a relatively small number of sampling units (PSUs) or counties; the 1999 sample was planned for only 12 PSUs. With a small number of PSUs, variance estimates

that account for the complex design will be relatively unstable, a factor which introduces a higher level of uncertainty in the annual estimates."

"Although the annual NHANES is nationally representative, it is not possible to produce environmental exposure estimates by geographic region. Because the number of geographic sites sampled each year is small and because environmental exposure measures may vary geographically, national estimates of these exposures, particularly those based on 1 year of data, may be highly variable."

"These limitations related to measuring environmental exposures from a single year of NHANES will be addressed as more data become available from the ongoing survey. More detailed analyses by demographic groups and other variables will be possible with increased sample size and with a larger number of geographic locations."

NCHS also raises the issue of the appropriateness of analyzing each phase of an NHANES separately in order to look for time trends. As noted in Section 9.0, NHANES-III was conducted in two consecutive phases. Each subject's participation in either the first or second phase is identified in the public database by the variable names of sdppsu1 and sdppsu2, and each phase has its own weighting factors. NCHS (1996b) indicates that:

"In NHANES III, 89 survey locations were randomly divided into two sets or phases, the first consisting of 44 and the other of 45 locations. One set of PSU's was allocated to the first three-year survey period (1988-91) and the other set to the second three-year period (1991-94). Therefore, unbiased national estimates of health and nutrition characteristics can be independently produced for each phase as well as for both phases combined. Computation of national estimates from both phases combined (i.e., total NHANES III) is the preferred option; individual phase estimates may be highly variable. In addition, individual phase estimates are not statistically independent. It is also difficult to evaluate whether differences in individual phase estimates are real or due to methodological differences. That is, differences may be due to changes in sampling methods or data collection methodology over time. At this time, there is no valid statistical test for examining differences between Phase 1 and Phase 2. Therefore, although point estimates can be produced separately for each phase, no test is available to test whether those estimates are significantly different from each other."

E) Issues of confidentiality.

In order to protect subject confidentiality, NCHS will not provide certain information (e.g., subject address or location, date of birth) with the publically available data. For example, in NHANES-III, NCHS identified the county of residence, but only if the county population exceeded 500,000. NCHS is even considering withholding some of the NHANES99+ biomonitoring data that were obtained from partial samples of the survey. Because of issues of confidentiality, it may be impossible to use the publicly available data to conduct some analyses that are of interest to EPA. For example, this would include studies in which it is necessary to know the location of the subjects and studies that need to link NHANES to other databases, such as exposure and mortality databases. Studies requiring confidential data should not be dismissed before contacting the NCHS RDC to determine if they are feasible if conducted through the Center (See Section 5.2 for details about conducting studies through the RDC).

F) Variable content within surveys.

In each of the NHANES, some variables (e.g., height, weight, age) are measured over the entire study and some are measured during only part of the survey. For example in NHANES-III, blood urea nitrogen was only measured in Phase II, but not in Phase I. Some variables are measured for all subjects (e.g., lead in blood was measured for all persons aged 1-74+ years in NHANES-III), and some variables are only measured for certain subgroups (e.g., allergy skin reactivity tests were administered to all persons aged 6-19 years and a random half-sample of the adults aged 20-59 years in NHANES-III). Some variables are measured for only a random sample within the survey (e.g., 1/3 of all subjects ages 12+ years have dioxins measured in serum for NHANES99+). Different data are collected for specific age groups and sometimes on the basis of gender (see Appendices IV, VI and VII). Note that as subjects get older, the number of chemicals tested in the blood and urine increases simply because the volume of body fluids that can be obtained increases. It is important to understand the variability in the content of a specific NHANES in order to design an analysis properly and to ensure that adequate numbers of subjects will be in each class or cell. Note that NCHS cautions against conducting an analysis with fewer than five subjects in a cell, as indicated by NCHS on their RDC website <http://www.cdc.gov/nchs/r&d/rdc.htm>. It is beyond the scope of this Handbook to provide a detailed discussion of this complicated survey design. The reader is referred to the following references for more complete discussions of the NHANES sample design. References for NHANES-I: NCHS (1973, 1977, 1978); for NHANES-II: NCHS(1981); for HHANES: NCHS (1985); for NHANES-III: NCHS (1994b, 1996c). The NCHS Documentation Books provide the counts of subjects for each variable measured in any survey. During the preliminary phases of designing a study, one can use these counts to determine if there are sufficient numbers of subjects to support the desired analysis. Documentation books can be downloaded for each survey from the following website <http://www.cdc.gov/nchs/about/major/nhanes/datalink.htm>.

G) Variable content and methods across surveys.

Given that data have been collected through NHANES for about 30 years and there are many variables that are measured across all the surveys, it may be intriguing to consider conducting some kind of time trend analyses. There are many precautions to consider before attempting such analyses, including the following: a) NHANES are cross-sectional studies and new subjects are recruited for each survey; b) While many variables have been measured across surveys, there is no guarantee that the measurement methods and equipment are the same and that test results are directly comparable. For example,

NHANES-I, -II and -III measured lung function by spirometry; however, each survey used different kinds of spirometers so it is not certain that lung function test results can be compared across surveys, or at least without some kind of adjustment. NCHS noted in their website <http://www.cdc.gov/nchs/about/major/nhanes/history.htm> that data collection for NHANES-II was made comparable to NHANES-I in order to establish a baseline for assessing changes over time. This means that in both surveys many of the same measurements were taken in the same way, on the same age segment of the U.S. population. A brief discussion of all NHANES can be found at the above noted website; c) Each survey is conducted at numerous locations throughout the U.S. (see Section 3.0) and the exact locations are not necessarily repeated from survey to survey. There are many variables (e.g., allergies, respiratory effects) that probably are affected by geographical location because of weather, altitude, humidity, degree of urbanization, pollution, etc. If you want to examine time trends, you will need to know which variables are sensitive to location of the subject and consider if this is going to be a problem; d) Differences in sample sizes and designs for each survey (see Sections 3.0, 4.0) must be considered when comparisons are made across the various surveys. For example, of the first four surveys, NHANES-III was the only survey that included persons 75 years or older, and NHANES- I and -II did not include any oversampling of Hispanics. Although the different surveys have similar analytic objectives, the differences in their sample sizes and designs will cause estimates to differ in reliability across the surveys (NCHS, 1996c).

9.0. ANALYSIS ISSUES

When analyzing NHANES data, it is important to take into account the complex survey design and the sample weights (see Sections 3, 4, and 8). Sample weights are needed to estimate means, medians, and other descriptive statistics. The weights must be used to produce correct population estimates because each SP does not have an equal probability of selection into the survey. The sample weights incorporate these differential probabilities of selection and include adjustments for noncoverage and nonresponse. Further, with the large oversampling of specific subgroups in each survey (e.g., young children, elderly, blacks, and Mexican-Americans in NHANES-III, also see Table 1), it is essential that sample weights be used in analyses, otherwise there is a risk that the results of the analysis will be incorrect. The data analysis must also take into account the strata and PSUs from the survey design used to estimate variances and test for statistical significance. In general, sampling variances will be underestimated if calculated without incorporating the complex survey design into the analysis (NCHS, 1994b).

Although preliminary analyses may be performed on unweighted data and with standard statistical packages that assume simple random sampling, the final analyses should be done on weighted data using special computer programs (e.g., SUDAAN, PCCARP) that employ appropriate methods for estimating variances from complex samples.

NCHS recently developed guidance for sample sizes needed to analyze complex survey data, such as NHANES (see Table 1 in Appendix I). This guidance takes into consideration

24

several issues, including the survey design and the rarity of the event (e.g., disease, physical condition) being studied.

9.1. Weighting

The purpose of weighting sample data is to permit analysts to produce estimates of statistics that would have been obtained if the entire sampling frame had been surveyed (NCHS, 1992b). The "sampling frame" is an operational definition of the target population, which in the case of NHANES is the civilian, non-institutionalized U.S. population. The specific definition of "entire sampling frame" varies among the individual NHANES surveys. For example, in NHANES-III, the entire sampling frame was the civilian, noninstitutionalized U.S. population ages two months and older. A sample weight can be thought of as the measure of the number of persons that a particular sample observation represents.

Each NHANES has its own set of weights and many are designed to accomplish the same objectives across the surveys. The reader should refer to NCHS (1975, 1982, 1992b and 1996c) for much more thorough discussions of how weights were computed for NHANES; how adjustments were made for non-response and poststratification; and how weights were calculated for specific survey components. To familiarize the reader with some of the issues involved in developing and using weights, the following information is provided based on the weighting used in NHANES-III; however, it is applicable to all of the surveys. Sample weighting in NHANES-III was used to accomplish the following objectives:

1) To compensate for differential probabilities of selection among subgroups. For example, members of different age-sex-race/ethnicity subgroups may be sampled at different rates and even oversampled. Persons living in different geographic regions also may be sampled at different rates;
2) To reduce biases arising from the fact that nonrespondents may be different from those who actually participate in the survey;
3) To bring sample data up to the dimensions of the target population totals (e.g., if one wants to use NHANES data to calculate national statistics, then the target population is the whole U.S. population);
4) To compensate, to the extent possible, for inadequacies in the sampling frame. These inadequacies may result from omissions of some housing units in the listing of area segments; omissions of persons with no fixed address, etc.; and
5) To reduce variances in the estimation procedure by using auxiliary information that is known with a high degree of accuracy.
(NCHS, 1996c and 1992b).

The procedure for weighting is summarized in the following paragraphs as presented in (NCHS, 1996c):

"The sample weighting was carried out in three stages. The first stage involved the computation of weights to compensate for unequal probabilities of selection (Objective 1 above). The second stage adjusted for nonresponse (Objective 2). The third stage used poststratification of the sample weights to Census Bureau estimates of the U.S. population to simultaneously accomplish the third, fourth, and fifth objectives. Due to the form of estimators typically used with data from complex samples, extreme variability in the weights may result in reduced reliability of the estimates. The NHANES-III sample was designed to minimize the variability in the weights, subject to operational and analytic constraints. When analyzing NHANES data, it is important to realize that extreme observations in conjunction with large weights may result in extremely influential observations, i.e., observations that dominate the analysis."

"If every selected household agreed to complete the screener questionnaire (to determine if eligible subjects lived in that house), and every selected person within the household agreed to complete the interview and the medical examination, then the weighted estimates based on the data would be close to unbiased estimates of statistics for the total U.S. population. However, nonresponse occurs in any survey operation, and nonresponse bias may result. All persons selected in the sample were asked to participate in a personal interview at their home, where medical history and socio-demographic information were collected. After the initial interview, all interviewed persons were invited to the MEC for a physical examination. Persons who were unable to come to the MEC were offered an abbreviated physical examination at their home (Note: this was only done in NHANES-III). Thus, nonresponse in NHANES can occur at several stages of the data collection process: a) some of the SPs who were screened refused to be interviewed (interview nonresponse); b) some of the interviewed SPs refused the medical examination (exam nonresponse); and c) some of the SPs participated at the MEC but refused specific tests."

"The issue of weighting is further complicated by the procedure of poststratification. Poststratification of sample weights to independent population estimates is used for several purposes. In most household surveys, certain demographic groups in the U.S. population (e.g., young black males) experience fairly high rates of undercoverage in survey efforts. Poststratification to Census estimates partially compensates for such undercoverage and for any differential nonresponse, and can help to reduce the resulting bias in the survey estimates. Poststratification can also help to reduce the variability of sample estimates as well as achieve consistency with accepted U.S. figures for various subpopulations, and bring the weighted totals up to the level of the presumed total civilian noninstitutionalized U.S. population."

As noted above from NCHS, 1996c, one needs to be aware of the important issue of large weights and particularly large weights in combination with extreme values (e.g., unusually high concentrations of pesticides in blood or urine of a specific subject). Either one of these conditions may unduly dominate the analysis and result in questionable, or inappropriate, conclusions. A good practice during the initial exploratory data phase would be to screen the weights to identify very large, influential values. It may also be useful to plot the values of the weights against the values of the analytes (e.g. concentrations of specific chemicals in blood and urine) to identify influential outliers. The results of these screening exercises should be used to help make a determination of how the observations associated with these weights should be handled in your analysis.

The following table, based on NHANES-III, illustrates the complexity of the survey weighting scheme, which includes not only overall interview and exam weights, but also weights for specific tests (e.g., allergy, and central nervous system (CNS)). NCHS survey documentation, which is part of the publicly available information, identifies the various weights and notes when it is appropriate to apply them.

Weight	Application
Final interview weight	Use only in conjunction with the sample interviewed at home, and only with items collected during the household interview.
Final exam (MEC only) weight	Use only in conjunction with the MEC examined sample, and only with interview and examination items collected at the MEC.
Final MEC+Home exam weight	Use only in conjunction with the MEC+Home examined sample, and only with items collected at both the MEC and home.
Final Allergy weight	Use only in conjunction with the Allergy subsample, and only with items collected as part of the allergy component of the exam.
Final CNS weight	Use only in conjunction with the CNS subsample, and only with items collected as part of the CNS component of the exam.
Final Standard exam (MEC only) weight	Use only in conjunction with the MEC examined persons assigned to the Standard subsample, and only with items collected at the MEC exam. These weights should be used to analyze tests such as the Oral Glucose Tolerance Tests (OGTT), where overnight fasting is preferred.
Final Modified exam (MEC only) weight	Use only in conjunction with the MEC examined persons assigned to the Modified subsample, and only with items collected at the MEC exam.
Final Standard MEC+Home exam weight	Use only in conjunction with the MEC and home examined persons assigned to the Standard subsample, and only with items collected during the MEC and home examinations.
Final Modified MEC+Home exam weight	Use only in conjunction with the MEC and home examined persons assigned to the Modified subsample, and only with items collected during the MEC and home examinations.

(NCHS, 1996c)

9.2. Issue of Nonresponse Bias

As noted above, nonresponse is a key issue with any survey, including NHANES. It is important to assess nonresponse bias in the analyses of data from complex samples such as NHANES. As indicated in NCHS (1994a), the assessment should include the following sections that focus on item nonresponse:

a) A definition of item nonresponse and the level of nonresponse;
b) A description of the effect of item nonresponse on statistics of interest;
c) Assumptions used in the adjustment methodology; and
d) An assessment of the imputation procedure and the impact of nonresponse adjustment on survey estimates.

NCHS (1994a) also notes that in addition to reporting nonresponse rates, to the extent possible, any analysis of nonresponse should include information on reasons for missing data (e.g., unable to contact subject, medical reasons, refusals, etc). Analysts should study the reasons for nonresponse at each stage of sampling. The researcher also needs to determine if the non-response is random or systematic. If there is systematic non-response by measured covariates (e.g., by specific demographic variables such as race/ethnicity or age), then the analyst needs to make an adjustment for it, for example, by reweighting the data. This information is valuable for diagnostic purposes in the evaluation of nonresponse bias.

It is beyond the scope of this Handbook to provide a detailed discussion of how to assesses and correct for subject nonresponse. The reader is referred to the following references for more complete discussions on how nonresponse is denoted in the surveys and how to adjust for nonresponse. For NHANES-I see NCHS(1973, 1977, 1978); NHANES-II see NCHS(1981); HHANES see NCHS(1985); NHANES-III see NCHS(1994a,b and 1996c).

10.0. SUMMARY AND CONCLUSIONS

This Handbook has provided a detailed overview of the purpose, history and content of NHANES; how to access the data and documentation; how NHANES data have been used by EPA and others to support public and environmental health studies and federal policies and regulations; and suggestions on how the data can be used in studies to support risk assessment, policy and regulatory needs at EPA. This document has also identified limitations and data analysis issues that need to be considered when designing a study using NHANES data. Despite the limitations and complex design of this survey, it is clear that NHANES is a unique, rich database that offers a tremendous amount of human health, nutrition, and exposure information, and will continue to do so into the future. Since the start of NHANES thirty years ago, EPA has participated in the design and support of each survey, but has only used the data for limited research, policy and regulatory needs. It is hoped that by informing staff about NHANES, this Handbook will encourage efforts to "mine" the data to support Agency needs across the Program Offices. It is also hoped that innovative approaches (e.g., using GIS; linking NHANES to available databases such as the National Death Index), will be tried in order to analyze the data in new ways that produce information that is useful to the mission of the Agency. Now that

NCHS has established their Research Data Center, it should be possible to conduct studies that were impossible in the past because of lack of access to sensitive data. Finally, more thought should be given to designing and conducting studies that make use of the subjects' biological samples (blood, urine, saliva) stored by NCHS. These samples offer a rare opportunity to study potential biomarkers of exposure and/or effects on a national sample of the U.S. population and to be able to link the data to health, nutrition, exposure and socioeconomic data already collected in the baseline surveys.

TABLE 1: Summary of Selected Design Features of the NHANES

SURVEY[a]	DATES of SURVEY	AGES EXAMINED	# OF SUBJECTS INTERVIEWED/ (EXAMINED)	NUMBER of SURVEY LOCATIONS (Stands)
NHANES-1[b]	1971-1975	1-74 years old	28,043/(20,739)	100
NHANES-II	1976-1980	6 mo.-74 years old	27,801/(20,322)	64
Hispanic HANES (HHANES)[c]	1982-1984	6 mo. -74 years old	15,931/(11,672)	17 in the southwest; 9 in NY, NJ, CT; 4 in FL
NHANES-III[d]	1988-1994	2 mo. +	39,695/(30,818)	89
NHANES99+[e]	started March 1999	all ages	5,000/yr.	15 per year

(Source: NCHS, 1994b; <http://www.cdc.gov/nchs/about/major/nhanes/current.htm>)

[a]Different surveys oversampled different subgroups as follows: NHANES-I, II (low income, children, elderly). NHANES-I also oversampled women ages 20-44 years. HHANES oversampled age groups 6mo.-19 yrs and 45-74 yrs old. NHANES III oversampled Black-Americans, Mexican-Americans, infants and young children (1-5 years) and older persons (60+ years).

[b] The first segment of NHANES-I was conducted from 1971-1974 and was followed by a 14 month period from 1974-1975 in which an additional national sample of people 25-74 years of age was examined to augment the size of the original sample. This additional sample is called the NHANES-I Augmentation Survey of Adults 25-74 years. (See <http://www.cdc.gov/nchs/data/series/sr_01/sr01_014.pdf> for more information)

[c]HHANES focused on the three largest Hispanic subgroups in the U.S.: Mexican-Americans in CA, AZ, NM, CO, TX; Cuban-Americans in Dade Co., FL; and Puerto Ricans in the New York City area. HHANES was conducted for two main reasons: 1) Hispanics were included in NHANES-I and II but not in sufficient numbers to produce estimates of the health of this ethnic group in general; and 2) NHANES-I and II did not collect specific data for Puerto Ricans, Mexican-Americans, or Cuban-Americans. HHANES was designed to produce estimates of the health and nutritional status of these three ethnic groups that were comparable to the estimates generated for the general population.

[d]NHANES-III had several unique features: 1) it was the first of these surveys to include infants 2 months of age and adults with no upper age limit; 2) it placed a greater emphasis on environmental health data, including testing ~1000 subjects for volatile organic compounds (VOCs) in their blood; and 3) it developed a home examination component for subjects who would not, or could not, go to the Mobile Examination Center (MEC). The home examination allowed for certain clinical tests that previously were only conducted at the MEC and this increased the number of data elements that were collected, primarily in elderly subjects. See Appendix IV for a summary of the NHANES-III examination and clinical biochemistry assessments and dietary/nutritional evaluations; and Appendix VII for a comparison of all the environmental data collected across the various NHANES.

[e]NHANES99+ continues to offer home examinations to subjects unable to go to the MEC.

Table 2. Summary of the NHANES-I Epidemiological Followup Studies

DATES of FOLLOWUP	AGES EXAMINED	NUMBER OF SPs	METHODS & DATA COLLECTED
Phase-I:1982- 84	all SPs 25-74 yrs old at baseline survey	14,407	face-to-face SP interview; pulse rate; weight; BP; self-reported conditions; hospital & nursing home records; death certificates
Phase-II: 1986	SPs 55-74 yrs old at baseline survey & not deceased at Phase-I	3,980	phone or mail interview; no physical measurements; hospital & nursing home records; death certificates
Phase-III: 1987	all non-deceased SPs	11,750	phone or mail interview; no physical measurements; hospital & nursing home records; death certificates
Phase-IV: 1991	all non-deceased SPs	11,195	interviews primarily by telephone; no physical measurements; health care facility abstracts; death certificates

(Sources: NCHS, 1987, 1990, 1992a, 1997)

Table 3. Schedule of Survey Planning Activities and Release of Data for NHANES-99 -08

Type of Activity	1999	2000	2001	2002	2003	2004	2005	2006	2007	2008
NHANES Planning Activities			Solicit proposals for 2003-2004	Pilot test new 2003-2004 components	Solicit proposals for 2005-2006	Pilot test new 2005-2006 components	Solicit proposals for 2007-2008	Pilot test new 2007-2008 components	Solicit proposals for 2009-2010	Pilot test new 2009-2010 components
NHANES Tabular Reports[1]		1999 Data release in 4th quarter		2001 Data release in 4th quarter	2002 Data release in 4th quarter	2003 Data release in 4th quarter	2004 Data release in 4th quarter	2005 Data release in 4th quarter	2006 Data release in 4th quarter	2007 Data release in 4th quarter
NHANES Micro-data Files				1999/2000 Release in 1st quarter		2001/2002 Release in 1st quarter		2003/2004 Release in 1st quarter		2005/2006 Release in 1st quarter
NHANES Dietary Data[2]				1999/2000 Release in 1st quarter		2001/2002 Release in 1st quarter[3]		2003/2004 Release in 1st quarter		2005/2006 Release in 1st quarter
NHANES Data Center Access[4]				Data years 1999 & 2000	2001 + earlier years	2002 + earlier years[5]	2003 +earlier years	2004 +earlier years	2005 +earlier years	2006 +earlier years
Survey	NHANES 1999-20000		NHANES 2001-2002		NHANES 2003-2004		NHANES 2005-2006		NHANES 2007-2008	

(Source: NHANES Consortium Meeting, 2002. This table was presented, as shown here, at this meeting.)
[1]Release of limited data tables on specific topics of public health significance. (Note: personal communication with NHCS staff indicated that tabular reports based on 2002 data would not be released.)

[2]Additional separate release of NHANES dietary recall data in accordance with DHHS/USDA survey integration plans.
[3]Without second day recall for 2002 to preserve confidentiality; USDA and HHS will work jointly to develop a bridging methodology to ensure comparability between data that is collected using different software and food composition data bases.
[4]NHANES variables not released on micro-data files due to disclosure risks. See information on NCHS Research Data Center and the NCHS Policy on Release of Micro Data.   [5]Includes second day dietary recall for 2002.

32

APPENDIX I

NHANES III Sample Design and Analysis Guidelines

(Note: The material in this Appendix is taken verbatim from the NCHS source document. A list of the references cited in the original NCHS document has not been included in this Appendix. The reader is referred to the source document for the full citations.)

(Source: NCHS, 1994b, pp.20-22)

SAMPLE DESIGN AND ANALYSIS GUIDELINES

Sample design

The general structure of the NHANES III sample design is the same as that of the previous NHANES. Each of these surveys used a stratified multistage probability design. The major design parameters of the two previous NHANES and the special Hispanic HANES, as well as NHANES III, have been previously summarized (17).

The NHANES III sample was designed to be self-weighting within a primary sampling unit (PSU) for subdomains and fairly close to self-weighting nationally for each of these subdomain groups (but not for the total population). The NHANES III sample represents the total civilian noninstitutionalized population, 2 months of age or over, in the 50 States of the United States. The first stage of the design consisted of selecting a sample of 81 PSU's, which, in the first stage, are mostly individual counties. In a few cases, adjacent counties were combined to keep PSU's above a minimum size. The PSU's were stratified and selected with probability proportional to size (PPS). Thirteen large counties (strata) were chosen with certainty (probability of one). For operational reasons, these 13 certainty PSU's were divided into 21 survey locations. After the 13 certainty strata were designated, the remaining PSU's in the United States were grouped into 34 strata, and 2 PSU's were selected per stratum (68 survey locations). The selection was done with PPS and without replacement. The NHANES III sample therefore consists of 81 PSU's or 89 locations.

The 89 stands were randomly divided into 2 sets, 1 consisting of 44 sites and the other 45 sites. One set of PSU's was allocated to the first 3-year survey period (1988–91) and the other set to the second 3-year period (1991–94). Therefore, unbiased estimates (from the point of view of sample selection) of health and nutrition characteristics can be independently produced for both Phase 1 and Phase 2 as well as for both phases combined.

For most of the sample, the second stage of the design consisted of area segments composed of city or suburban blocks, combinations of blocks, or other area segments in places where block statistics were not produced in the 1980 census. In the first phase of NHANES III, the area segments were used only for a sample of persons who lived in housing units built before 1980. For units built in 1980 and later, the second stage consisted of sets of addresses selected from building permits issued in 1980 or later. These are referred to as ''new construction segments.'' In the second phase, 1990 census data and maps were used to define the area segments. Because the second phase followed within a few years of the 1990 census, new construction did not account for a significant part of the sample and the entire sample came from the area segments.

The third stage of sample selection consisted of households and certain types of group quarters, such as dormitories. All households and eligible group quarters in the sample segments were listed, and a subsample was designated for screening in order to identify potential sample persons. The subsampling rates enabled production of a national, approximately equal, probability sample of households in most of the United States, with higher rates for the geographic strata with high Mexican-American populations. Within each geographic stratum, there is an approximate equal-probability sample of households across all 89 stands. The screening rate in each stratum was designed to produce the desired number of sample persons for the rarest age-sex domain in the race and ethnic group defining the geographic stratum.

Persons within the sample of households or group quarters were the fourth stage of sample selection. All eligible members within a household were listed, and a subsample of individuals was selected based on sex, age, and race or ethnicity. The definitions of the sex, age, race or ethnic classes, subsampling rates, and designation of potential sample persons within screened households were developed to provide approximately self-weighting samples for each subdomain within geographic strata and at the same time to maximize the average number of sample persons per sample household. Experience in previous NHANES indicated that this increased the overall participation rate. Although the exact sample sizes will not be known until data collection has been completed, estimates have been made. A summary of the expected sample sizes at each stage of the design is as follows:

Number of PSU's	81
Number of stands (survey locations)	89
Number of segments	2,138
Number of households to be screened	106,000
Number of households with sample persons	20,000
Number of sample persons	40,600
Number of interviewed sample persons	35,000
Number of examined sample persons	30,100

A more detailed description of the sample design for NHANES III, including a description of the research that resulted in the final design, has been previously published (17).

Analysis guidelines

Because of the complex survey design used in NHANES III, traditional methods of statistical analysis based on the assumption of a simple random sample are not applicable. Detailed descriptions of this issue and possible analytic methods for analyzing NHANES data have been described previously (7,79,134,135). These previously recommended guidelines are revised on a periodic basis as new statistical procedures and analytic computer software are developed. However, there are some important analysis considerations that have not changed over time.

First, there are the two aspects of the NHANES design that must be taken into account in data analysis. One is the sample weights and the other is the complex survey design. Sample weights are needed to estimate means, medians, and other descriptive statistics. They must be used to produce correct population estimates because each sample person does not have an equal probability of selection. The sample weights incorporate these differential probabilities of selection and include adjustments for noncoverage and nonresponse. With the large oversampling of young children, older persons, black persons, and Mexican-Americans in NHANES III, it is essential that the sample weights be used in all analyses. Otherwise, misinterpretation of results is highly likely.

The second aspect of the design that must be taken into account in data analysis is the strata and PSU's from the sample design used to estimate variances and test for statistical significance. In general, sampling variances will be underestimated if calculated without incorporating the complex sample design.

The effect of the complex sample design on variance estimates is referred to as the design effect, which is the ratio of the variance of a statistic from a complex sample to the variance of the same statistic from a simple random sample of the same size (3). A design effect of one indicates the equality of the simple random sample variance and the complex sample variance.

Design effects in NHANES have traditionally been higher than one, and the magnitude of the design effects have been variable. In NHANES I and NHANES II, the average design effect was calculated to be about 1.5. Preliminary analyses from NHANES III indicate that the average design effect might be lower (approximately 1.2 or 1.3).

Although preliminary analyses may be performed on unweighted data with standard statistical packages that assume simple random sampling, final analyses should be done on weighted data using special computer programs that use an appropriate method for estimating variances from a complex sample (e.g., SUDAAN (136) or PCCARP (137)). The calculation and use of "average" design effects (when unstable variances occur) along with the sample weights have been suggested as an alternative NHANES analytic approach (135). Recently, NCHS staff have participated in an effort to establish guidelines for variance estimation and statistical reporting standards. In addition to delineating some of the previously mentioned issues, the staff produced a nomogram of recommended sample sizes for analyses of complex survey data (table 1). For means of fairly symmetric populations and proportions based on commonly occurring events (where $0.25 < p < 0.75$), a good rule of thumb is that the sample size should be no smaller than some broadly calculated "average design effect" times 30. The first column of the table represents a simple random sample design and the other columns reflect the increased sample size requirements for a more complex survey design. Thus, the minimum sample size for a normal approximation increases for more rare events as well as for survey designs that result in increased average design effects. Other criteria and approaches for estimating minimum sample sizes exist; however, this is the approach currently proposed for NHANES III analyses.

Table 1. Recommended sample sizes for a complex survey design, by design effect and specified proportion

Proportion	Design effect													
	1.0	1.1	1.2	1.3	1.4	1.5	1.6	1.7	1.8	1.9	2.0	2.5	3.0	3.5
0.99	800	880	960	1,040	1,120	1,200	1,280	1,360	1,440	1,520	1,600	2,000	2,400	2,800
0.95	160	176	192	208	224	240	256	272	288	304	320	400	480	560
0.90	80	88	96	104	112	120	128	136	144	152	160	200	240	280
0.85	53	59	64	69	75	80	85	91	96	101	107	133	160	187
0.80	40	44	48	52	56	60	64	68	72	76	80	100	120	140
0.75	32	35	38	42	45	48	51	54	58	61	64	80	96	112
0.56–0.74	30	33	36	39	42	45	48	51	54	57	60	75	90	105
0.55	30	33	36	39	42	45	48	51	54	57	60	75	90	105
0.50	30	33	36	39	42	45	48	51	54	57	60	75	90	105
0.45	30	33	36	39	42	45	48	51	54	57	60	75	90	105
0.26–0.44	30	33	36	39	42	45	48	51	54	57	60	75	90	105
0.25	32	35	38	42	45	48	51	54	58	61	64	80	96	112
0.20	40	44	48	52	56	60	64	68	72	76	80	100	120	140
0.15	53	59	64	69	75	80	85	91	96	101	107	133	160	187
0.10	80	88	96	104	112	120	128	136	144	152	160	200	240	280
0.05	160	176	192	208	224	240	256	272	288	304	320	400	480	560
0.01	800	880	960	1,040	1,120	1,200	1,280	1,360	1,440	1,520	1,600	2,000	2,400	2,800

Note: Minimum sample size requirements are adjusted for the relative inefficiency in the sample design by a factor equal to the design effect where design effect = complex sample variance/simple random sample variance
For midrange proportions (0.25 <p<0.75), the simple random sample (SRS) minimum sample size is 30.
For extreme proportions (≤0.25 or p≥0.75), the SRS sample size (n) satisfies the following rule: n(p)≥8 and n(1-p)≥8.

I-5

These guidelines reflect a design-based approach to estimation and analysis. In some instances, a model-based approach may be used. The use of an "average design effect" to estimate the complex sample variances is one such instance. The use of model-based approaches is most appropriate when maximizing use of all available data is preferable (138,139).

It is important to remember that guidelines are just that, and they are not absolutes. They represent strategies that yield the most sound statistical conclusions. Violating the guidelines introduces a greater degree of uncertainty about the soundness of the analytic conclusions but does not necessarily mean that a particular analysis is invalid. Consideration of the survey design, survey nonresponse, data collection and processing procedures, potential measurement errors, and the subject matter being studied are all equally important and should be evaluated to judge the merit of each analysis and interpretation of data from any survey, including NHANES III.

APPENDIX II

NHANES III Health Status Assessment

(Note: The material in this Appendix is taken verbatim from the NCHS source document. A list of the references cited in the original NCHS document has not been included in this Appendix. The reader is referred to the source document for the full citations.)

(Source: NCHS, 1994b, pp. 3-13)

HEALTH STATUS ASSESSMENT

Because of the variety and complexity of the data collected in NHANES III, the information in this section is presented in different ways. The first part provides overviews of some of the main areas of special interest addressed in NHANES III and highlights some of the public health and scientific issues covered by the survey in each of these areas. The second part provides a more detailed account of the data collected by examination and interview for each of the major health topic areas included in the survey. The third part describes the risk factors and health behaviors measured in NHANES III, and the fourth part describes three special studies.

Health of population subgroups and topics of special interest

In this section some of the major contributions made by NHANES III in assessing and monitoring the health of population subgroups of interest, including children and adolescents, the elderly, women, and minorities, are described. Also covered are contributions in providing information on special topics, including environmental and occupational health and the assessment of health care coverage and needs. NHANES III is a national survey, designed to collect information to assess the health status of the entire U.S. civilian, noninstitutionalized population. Within that framework, however, the survey was also designed to sample large numbers of young children, older persons, black persons, and Mexican- Americans, so that reliable estimates of health status can be produced for these population subgroups.

Child and adolescent health

NHANES III is the first NHANES to include children as young as 2 months of age. The survey was designed to oversample children aged 2 months to 5 years so new growth charts could be created for use in assessing children's growth and development. To increase the response rates among infants aged 2–11 months, the option of a home examination was offered to parents unwilling to bring very young children to the mobile examination center (MEC).

NHANES III data on child health are relevant to many key areas of public health for children in the United States. Environmental lead exposure and progress in reducing children's lead exposure were assessed by questionnaire data and measurements of blood lead levels for all children 1 year of age and over. Information on children's exposure to tobacco smoke was gained by questionnaire data on smoking by household members, coupled with measurement of serum cotinine levels. Measurements of hepatitis B markers, tetanus antitoxin, diphtheria antibody, and rubella antibody levels serve to assess and monitor immunization levels in children. The use of NHANES III data in the creation of new growth charts is discussed in more detail in the section "Nutritional health assessment." Also relevant to child health is the knowledge gained from NHANES III about the health status of women of childbearing age, including folate status and susceptibility to the rubella virus.

The content of the survey varied for children of different ages. However, in general, for infants and young children (2 months to 5 years of age), the survey included information on oral health, growth, and motor and social development. For older children and adolescents, NHANES III collected data on varied conditions that include asthma and allergy, pulmonary function, oral health, hearing, cognitive function, blood pressure, and stage of sexual maturation as well as questionnaire data on physical activity and tobacco use and many laboratory determinations. In addition, adolescents were asked in private interviews about tobacco, drug, and alcohol use, reproductive history, and mental health.

Health of older persons

NHANES III is the first NHANES to include persons 75 years of age and over. In order to address scientific and policy issues pertinent to the older population in the United States, NHANES III included an oversample of older persons (aged 60 years and over). To minimize nonresponse in older persons, a home examination was developed for those persons who were unable or unwilling to come to the MEC for a complete examination. This home examination included an abbreviated set of measures parallel to those performed in the MEC.

The survey content of NHANES III is particularly useful for the study of the contribution of multiple diseases to disability in old age. As covered in other sections of this report, this content included nutritional status, cardiovascular disease, pulmonary disease, dental disease, diabetes, retinopathy, osteoarthritis, and osteoporosis. Besides these specific diseases, the survey included measures of functional status in older persons to ascertain the prevalence of disability and limitations in function and the correlations of patterns of disease with functional health status.

The survey addressed three major areas of function: social, cognitive, and physical function. Much of the content of NHANES III in these areas was shaped by a special workshop, "Innovations in the Measurement of Function for Older Persons: A Focus on National Surveys," held in September 1985.

Minority health

NHANES III is the first NHANES to include planned oversampling of the two largest minority groups in the United States. The black and Mexican-American populations were oversampled to obtain statistically reliable estimates for the two largest minority groups in the United States. In previous national surveys, although these groups were included in the sample according to their representation in the national population, sample sizes were often too small to provide adequate estimates. As a result, it was decided to include planned oversampling of these two groups in NHANES III.

The content of the examination is targeted to the national population as a whole and to specific age ranges, rather than to specific minority groups. However, many health conditions studied in the survey occur at high rates in minority populations, including diabetes mellitus among Mexican-Americans and hypertension among black persons. The survey provides extensive data for minorities on chronic diseases, renal function, pulmonary function, environmental exposures, immunization status, risk factors, and health behaviors. In addition, because the survey included oversampling of children and the elderly, NHANES III provides information on the health of black and Mexican-American children and older persons. In many of these areas, NHANES III provides the first comprehensive national data and reference standards for the black and Mexican-American populations. Further, NHANES III data allow for valid comparisons among different race-ethnic groups because data were collected in a standardized manner for all survey participants. Race-ethnic groups were defined based upon combinations of the reported race and reported ethnicity of survey participants. These data can be used to provide insight into the causes and concomitants of the disparities in health status among race-ethnic groups in the United States.

Women's health

Women's health has traditionally referred primarily to issues related to reproduction. In recent years there has been a heightened awareness that women's health encompasses a wide range of conditions, for many of which adequate data are lacking. Although NHANES III does not include oversampling of the female population, it was designed to include equal numbers of males and females in each age and race ethnic subgroup. Thus the survey provides extensive data on the health status of girls and women in the United States. Because the survey included special emphasis on the health of older persons, as well as oversampling of minority populations, data will be available on older women and on black and Mexican-American women. Many of the components in NHANES III were also included in previous surveys, allowing study of trends over time.

The survey content includes extensive information on reproductive health as well as on many conditions that are either of high prevalence in women or that occur more frequently in women than in men. These conditions include cardiovascular disease, the leading cause of death in women (18), osteoporosis, diabetes, arthritis, thyroid dysfunction, obesity, gallbladder disease, and mental conditions.

Environmental and occupational health

NHANES III provides new national population data relevant to occupational and environmental health. Markers of exposure to toxic metals and assessments reflecting indoor air quality were the focus of the environmental health data collected in the survey. These activities were, in part, a response to Title IV (Radon Gas and Indoor Air Quality Research) of the Superfund Amendments and Reauthorization Act of 1986 (Public Law 99–499).

In NHANES III, blood lead level, a key indicator of exposure to environmental lead, was measured for the second time in the U.S. population. NHANES II (1976–80) lead data were used extensively to assess the extent of exposure to lead in the United States, to identify correlates of exposure (e.g., urbanization, age), to monitor trends in exposure, to support policy and regulatory decisions regarding lead in gasoline, and to identify health effects resulting from lead exposure (e.g., blood pressure elevations, diminished height in children) (19). It is expected that the lead data from NHANES III will serve a similar purpose during the 1990's. Cadmium, a toxicologic concern ranking close to that of lead (20), was measured for the first time in NHANES III.

In 1985, the Interagency Committee for Indoor Air Quality identified NHANES III as providing an important opportunity to examine the relation of indoor pollutant exposures to potential health effects on a national basis (21). Although levels of indoor air pollutants were not directly measured in the NHANES III homes, data were collected on housing characteristics, water sources, and cooking and heating fuel systems. Information on health outcomes related to the indoor environment included data on respiratory symptoms and smoking history, measurements of allergic reactivity to mites (house dust), pulmonary function testing, and the physician's assessment of bronchial sounds. Tobacco smoke is a significant indoor air pollutant, and passive exposure to tobacco smoke has been determined to be a major health hazard by the Environmental Protection Agency (22). In NHANES III, serum cotinine levels were measured to determine active and passive exposure to tobacco smoke and other sources of nicotine.

A report by the House Committee on Government Operations entitled "Occupational Health Hazard Surveillance—72 Years Behind and Counting" (23) provided the impetus for the NHANES III collection of more data related to occupational health. Three examination components were designed to assess potential health effects that may result from occupational exposure: the neurobehavioral evaluation system (NES) for central nervous system testing, the physician's examination for assessing hand blistering and redness, and the spirometry test for measuring pulmonary function. Questions on current and longest held occupation, use of protective equipment at work and passive exposure to smoke at work were also included.

Health care coverage and health care needs

NHANES III provides a unique opportunity to assess the prevalence of unrecognized disease and unmet health care needs. Because this is an examination survey, it allows for objective determination by examination and measurement of many health conditions. Thus it is possible to assess the degree to which these conditions are recognized and the implications for health care needs.

For example, NHANES III measurements of blood pressure, combined with information on prior diagnosis and on the use of antihypertension medications or nonpharmacologic therapy can be used to estimate the extent to which persons with high blood pressure are aware of their condition, the extent to which those who are aware are receiving treatment, and the extent to which those receiving treatment have reduced their blood pressure to acceptable levels. National data on blood cholesterol levels from NHANES III were used to estimate the numbers of people requiring intervention and treatment under the Adult Treatment Panel guidelines of the National Cholesterol Education Program and to monitor changes since similar data were collected in NHANES II. Dental examination data can be used to describe the extent of population needs for dental care, the extent to which existing conditions have been treated, and, coupled with information on dental care utilization, the degree of access to dental care for people with differing needs. Immunization data obtained from blood samples can be used to assess the level of protection in the population.

As part of NHANES III, data on health care utilization, health insurance coverage for all family members, and income assistance, including Medicaid, Social Security, and Supplemental Security Income, were collected to assess health care needs and participation in public assistance programs. Participants were asked detailed questions about coverage by Medicare, other forms of health insurance or reasons for lack of coverage, and about their use of health services and medications, established relationships with providers, and history of health conditions and hospitalizations. These data can be used in conjunction with the other information collected in the survey to determine the relationships between access to care and health status.

Health status components

This part provides a brief account of the data collected by examination and interview for each of the major target conditions and physiological measurements in NHANES III. In the survey, data were collected on dietary intake and nutritional status (described in the section "Nutritional health assessment''), anthropometric measurements (described in that same section), reproductive history and sexual behaviors, use of vitamin and mineral supplements and medications, tobacco and alcohol use, physical activity, and sociodemographic characteristics. These data, although not mentioned specifically, are relevant to many of the components. A list of topics included in the questionnaires administered during the household interview and in the questionnaires and procedures administered in the examination can be found in appendix tables I and II. Other summary information is included in appendix I and appendix tables III–XII and the data collection forms are in appendixes III and IV.

The examination teams, described more fully in the section "Data collection and reports of findings," included a physician, a dentist, a certified ultrasound technician, health technicians, medical technologists, a phlebotomist, a health interviewer, and dietary interviewers, as well as other personnel. Except as noted under specific components, a health technician administered all MEC examination procedures, and the health interviewer administered the MEC adult, youth, and proxy questionnaires. Examinees were excluded from each of the examination components for specific safety, health, or logistical reasons. These exclusion criteria are specified in appendix table VIII.

Fasting instructions were common to all components. For morning examinations, examinees aged 12–19 years were instructed to fast at least 8.5 hours preceding the examination, and those 20 years of age and over were instructed to fast 12 hours. For afternoon or evening examinations, all examinees 12 years of age and over were instructed to fast for 6 hours preceding the examination. Children under age 12 and persons of any age who reported using insulin were instructed not to fast.

Many laboratory determinations were conducted on blood and urine specimens obtained during the MEC examination. Most of these determinations are mentioned briefly under the relevant topic headings. However, the laboratory methods are not described in any detail in this section. Full procedural descriptions of the laboratory methods are available from NCHS, and a summary of the assay methods is provided in appendix I. For the convenience of the reader, the laboratory analyses conducted in all three of the NHANES and the Hispanic HANES are provided in appendix table VI. A complete list of all the laboratory determinations on blood and urine specimens can be found in appendix table IV. The laboratories and diagnostic centers are also listed in appendix table III.

Cardiovascular disease

Cardiovascular disease, including coronary heart disease and stroke, is the leading cause of death in the United States for both men and women (18). Since the first National Health Examination Survey in 1960–62, the assessment of cardiovascular disease-related risk factors and, to a lesser extent, cardiovascular disease have been a central component of the NHANES program (1). The main elements of the cardiovascular disease component in NHANES III were measurements of blood pressure, measurements of blood lipid levels, and electrocardiograms (ECG's).

For the first time in any NHANES, blood pressure was measured on two separate occasions to reduce misclassification error. For adults 17 years of age and over, a total of six seated blood pressure measurements were obtained: three by the interviewer in the household interview and three by the physician during the MEC examination. For children 5–16 years of age, three blood pressure measurements were made in the MEC by the physician. In the MEC, the first, fourth, and fifth Korotkoff sounds (K1, K4, and K5) were recorded for those 5–19 years of age, and K1 and K5 were recorded for those 20 years of age and over. Blood pressure measurements were conducted according to the standardized measurement protocols recommended by the American Heart Association (24).

ECG's were done on all examinees 40 years of age and over. The ECG's were interpreted by computer using the Minnesota Code (25). The physician's examination in the MEC included assessment of systolic and diastolic heart murmurs for all examinees.

Blood lipid levels were determined on a specimen obtained by venipuncture during the MEC or home examination. Serum total cholesterol, high-density lipoprotein (HDL) cholesterol, and serum triglycerides were measured on all examinees 4 years of age and over. Measurements of total and HDL cholesterol and fasting triglyceride levels permit low-density lipoprotein (LDL) cholesterol levels to be calculated using the equation developed by Friedewald, Levy, and Fredrickson (26). Phase 1 of the survey also included measurements of apolipoproteins A1 and B, and Phase 2 included measurements of Lp(a), both for all examinees 4 years of age and over.

The Household Adult Questionnaire, administered to adults aged 17 years and over, included questions on family history of heart attack; history, knowledge, and treatment of high blood pressure and high blood cholesterol; and history of heart attack, stroke, transient ischemic attacks, and congestive heart failure. The questionnaire also included three sections from the London School of Hygiene Cardiovascular Questionnaire (27), including the Rose Angina, Possible Infarction, and Intermittent Claudication questions. During the household interview, the interviewer made three seated blood pressure measurements (K1 and K5) for adults aged 17 years and over.

The Household Youth Questionnaire included questions on history of rheumatic fever and heart disease for children aged 2 months to 16 years and questions on history of high blood pressure and high blood cholesterol for children aged 4–16 years.

Respiratory disease

Respiratory disease has a substantial effect on morbidity and mortality rates in the United States. It is estimated that up to 20 percent of the adult population suffer from one of the chronic obstructive pulmonary diseases (asthma, chronic bronchitis, or emphysema) (28).

The respiratory disease component for NHANES III was designed to measure pulmonary function and chronic obstructive pulmonary disease. The main element of the component was assessment of pulmonary function by spirometry. Respondents were also tested for skin-test reactivity to selected standardized allergens.

Spirometry was conducted for all examinees 8 years of age and over in the MEC or home examinations. Procedures for testing were based on the current recommendations and standards of the American Thoracic Society (29). A customized Ohio Censored 822 or 827 dry rolling seal spirometer was used in the MEC and a portable spirometer was used in the home examination. Examinees performed five to eight blows to obtain curves acceptable according to the protocol. The National Institute for Occupational Safety and Health (NIOSH) was responsible for training the technicians, providing the equipment, and processing the spirometry data.

The Household Adult Questionnaire, administered to adults 17 years of age and over, included questions on the medical history of respiratory and allergic symptoms and conditions. Additional questions ascertained previous diagnosis of asthma, chronic bronchitis, or emphysema. The Household Youth Questionnaire included a similar set of questions for children aged 2 months to 16 years.

Diabetes mellitus

Diabetes mellitus is well recognized as a major public health problem in the United States. The disease affects virtually every organ system in the body, and the rates of such conditions as kidney disease, blindness, hypertension, ischemic heart disease, stroke, and disability are significantly higher in persons with diabetes. The direct and indirect costs of diabetes in the United States were estimated to be more than $20 billion in 1987 (30), and diabetes ranks as the seventh leading cause of death (18).

The diabetes component was designed to assess glucose tolerance and diabetes. The main elements of the component were an oral glucose tolerance test and other diabetes-related laboratory determinations. Related information includes the data collected in the diabetic retinopathy and vision component.

The MEC examination included a 2-hour 75-gram oral glucose tolerance test (OGTT). Adults 40–74 years of age examined in the morning session were given the OGTT after being instructed to fast for 12 hours prior to the examination. After a fasting blood specimen was obtained by venipuncture, examinees were then administered a glucose challenge (Dextol- 75) containing the equivalent of 75 grams of glucose. A second blood specimen was drawn 2 hours after the fasting blood specimen. Measurements of fasting and 2-hour plasma glucose levels permit identification of diabetes and impaired glucose tolerance according to World Health Organization (WHO) criteria (31).

Adults 40–74 years of age who were examined in the afternoon or evening were given the OGTT after being instructed to fast for 6 hours prior to the examination. This procedure does not follow exactly the WHO recommendations. However, the National Diabetes Data Group of the National Institute of Diabetes and Digestive and Kidney Diseases strongly recommended that all adult participants 40–74 years of age be screened for glucose tolerance in order to have sufficient numbers of subjects to ascertain the natural history of glucose intolerance and to quantify risk factors for the development of diabetes.

Fasting blood specimens obtained by venipuncture during the MEC examination from adults 20 years of age and over were tested for glucose, levels of insulin, and C-peptide. Glycated hemoglobin concentration (Hb_{A1c}) was determined in all individuals 4 years of age and over as a measure of glucose levels over time. In Phase 2, insulin and C-peptide levels were also measured on the 2-hour blood specimens for adults 40–74 years of age. The Household Adult Questionnaire, administered to adults aged 17 years and over, included questions designed to ascertain those individuals with a medical history of diabetes. Information collected included family history and age at diagnosis; use, frequency, and amount of insulin taken; use of oral hypoglycemic agents or diet to lower blood glucose levels; and reported retinopathy. The Household Youth Questionnaire included questions on diabetes and insulin use for safety screening purposes only.

Diabetic retinopathy and vision

The diabetic retinopathy and vision component of NHANES III was designed to assess diabetic retinopathy and macular degeneration, two of the major causes of severe visual handicap and blindness among adults in the United States (32). The main element of the component was retinal photography carried out in the MEC. Related information includes the data collected in the diabetes component.

The MEC examination included a nonmydriatic fundus photograph of either the right or left eye for all examinees 40 years of age and over (33–35). The eye to be photographed was randomly selected according to the last digit of the examinee's identification number. Photographic fields were graded by masked, trained graders for macular degeneration, for the presence and severity of retinopathy and for the presence of specified diabetic lesions using the Modified Airlie House Classification scheme (36). The training of photographers and the grading of photographic slides was done by the staff of the Department of Ophthalmology, University of Wisconsin Medical School.

In the physician's examination, examinees aged 2 months to 18 years were evaluated for a missing globe or blindness; children 2 months–4 years of age were examined for ability to track light; and those 5–18 years of age were examined for strabismus. No funduscopic examination was included in the physician's examination and no vision examination was included in the survey.

The Household Adult Questionnaire, administered to adults 17 years of age and over, included questions on problems with vision and presence of blindness, cataracts, or retinopathy. The Household Youth Questionnaire included an abbreviated set of vision questions for children aged 2 months–16 years.

Thyroid function

The thyroid component of NHANES III was designed to provide information on the prevalence of autoimmune thyroid disease, thyroid function, iodine intake, and population estimates for normal hormone levels through laboratory measurements.

Measurement of serum thyroid-stimulating hormone (TSH), thyroxine (T4), and antithyroglobulin and antimicrosomal antibodies were conducted on blood specimens obtained by venipuncture during the MEC examination from examinees 12 years of age and over. Urinary iodine and creatinine were also measured for examinees 12 years of age and over to evaluate the relationship between iodine intake and thyroid dysfunction.

The Household Adult Questionnaire, administered to adults aged 17 years and over, included questions regarding history of goiter or other thyroid diseases.

Reproductive health

The reproductive health component of NHANES III was composed of questions on the menstrual cycle, pregnancy history, menopause, use of contraception, and sexual experience among women, as well as laboratory determinations of follicle-stimulating hormone (FSH), luteinizing hormone (LH), and pregnancy and lactation status. Related information includes data collected in the immunization and infectious disease component.

In the MEC Proxy Questionnaire, data were collected on age of menarche for girls 8–9 years of age. In the MEC Youth Questionnaire, girls 10–16 years of age were asked about age of menarche and were asked to estimate the time since their last period. Girls aged 12–16 years were asked about pregnancy history, breast feeding, use of oral contraceptives, and sexual experience. In the MEC Adult Questionnaire, women 17 years of age and over were asked about age at menarche, pregnancy history, breast feeding, natural and surgical menopause, use of NORPLANT, use of estrogen, sexual experience, and whether they had ever had genital herpes. A similar set of reproductive history questions was included in the home examination for women 20 years of age and over.

FSH and LH levels were determined on blood specimens obtained by venipuncture during the MEC examination from women 35–60 years. In addition, a urine pregnancy test was administered in the MEC to women 20–59 years of age.

Kidney disease

Kidney diseases constitute a major public health problem with rapidly increasing visibility because of the fast-growing numbers of patients with end stage renal disease (ESRD). The number of patients enrolled in the Medicare ESRD program increased from 113,542 in 1984 to more than 170,000 in 1989 (37). The annual costs of the ESRD program have continued to increase since 1974. The annual expenditures for 1974 were reported to be $229 million and had reached almost $3 billion in 1989 for this program (38). Based on both the escalating costs and increasing numbers of patients being served by the ESRD program, cost-effective preventive measures must be implemented.

The kidney disease component of the NHANES III was designed to assess renal function. The main elements of the component were laboratory determinations on blood and urine specimens. Urinary albumin (microalbuminuria) and creatinine levels were measured in urine specimens collected during the MEC examination from examinees aged 6 years and over. Measurements of serum creatinine and blood urea nitrogen (BUN) were made on blood specimens obtained by venipuncture from examinees 12 years of age and over. The Household Adult Questionnaire, administered to adults aged 17 years and over, included questions on the history of kidney and urologic disorders.

Gallstone disease

Approximately 600,000 patients undergo cholecystectomy each year, making it the most common abdominal surgical procedure. As a cause of hospitalization, gallstone disease is the most common and most costly digestive disease, with an annual overall cost of well over $5 billion (39).

The gallbladder component for the NHANES III was designed to determine the prevalence of diagnosed and undiagnosed gallstone disease. The main element of the component was real-time ultrasonography, a noninvasive technique for detecting gallstones. The ultrasound examination of the gallbladder was administered by a certified abdominal ultrasound technician to all examinees 20–74 years of age. Examinations were conducted with examinees in both supine and left decubitus positions. A diagnosis of gallstone disease was made by commonly used criteria of echoes within the gallbladder with shadowing in two views. Diagnoses were first made by the ultrasound technician in the MEC and later confirmed by radiologists. If a right upper quadrant or epigastric scar was observed and the gallbladder was not seen, it was concluded that a cholecystectomy had been performed. Data for other abnormal pathologies observed in the surrounding areas, such as the liver or the right kidney, were also recorded.

The Household Adult Questionnaire, administered to adults 17 years of age and over, included questions on previous diagnosis of gallstone disease, surgery for gallstones, or other gallbladder disease. Further questions ascertained occurrence, frequency, and character of pain in the abdomen or lower chest.

Arthritis and related musculoskeletal conditions

Arthritis and related musculoskeletal disorders are frequently chronic, disabling, and painful. It is estimated that the total economic cost to the United States of musculoskeletal conditions was more than $126 billion in 1988 (40).

The arthritis component of NHANES III was designed to identify rheumatoid arthritis and osteoarthritis in adults 60 years of age and over. The main elements of the component were radiographs and physician's examination of joints. Related information includes data collected in the osteoporosis and functional health status of the elderly components.

During the MEC examination, straight posterior-anterior x rays of the hands and wrists and straight anterior-posterior non-weight-bearing views of the knees were obtained for examinees aged 60 years and over. The knee position was selected because of safety considerations related to the space limitations in the MEC. Additional data were collected during the physician's examination for those 60 years of age and over. Hand, knee, and great toe joints were examined for tenderness, swelling, and pain on passive motion. The presence of hand and foot deformities was also recorded. Abnormalities in gait were evaluated by the physician for all examinees 3 years of age and over.

Serologic analyses of rheumatoid factor for examinees aged 60 years and over and of C-reactive protein for examinees 4 years of age and over were conducted on blood obtained by venipuncture during the MEC examination.

The Household Adult Questionnaire, administered to adults 17 years of age and over, included questions on joint pain, stiffness and swelling in hands, wrists, and knees, back pain, and medical history of arthritis.

Osteoporosis

The growing recognition of the public health significance of osteoporosis coupled with the lack of prevalence estimates based on a nationally representative sample motivated the inclusion of the osteoporosis component in NHANES III. The cost of hip fractures was estimated to be $3.5 billion per year in the United States (41). Those who survive hip fracture are often permanently disabled and must be institutionalized. The extent of problems associated with hip fracture is likely to increase in the future as the population ages, so that the number of hip fractures may double or triple by the year 2050 (42). The NHANES osteoporosis component was designed to assess many of the suspected risk factors for osteoporosis and hip fracture in a nationally representative sample of adults over 20 years of age.

Although osteoporosis cannot currently be defined by bone density alone, low bone density is a primary risk factor for osteoporotic fracture, with the risk of fracture increasing as bone density decreases (43, 44). The cornerstone of the osteoporosis component was the measurement of bone density at the proximal femur of adults 20 years of age and over. Related information includes data collected in the functional health status of the elderly and arthritis and related musculoskeletal conditions components. Several bone-related biochemistries were also measured.

Bone density measurements were made with dual-energy x-ray absorptiometry or DXA (45). The equipment measured areal bone density (bone mass per unit of area scanned) in five regions of interest in the proximal femur: femoral neck, trochanter, intertrochanter, Ward's triangle, and total region. Scans were reviewed by consultants at the Mayo Clinic for the purpose of quality control.

The Household Adult Questionnaire, administered to adults aged 17 years and over, included an extensive series of questions on history of falls and fractures and on maternal history of fractures and osteoporosis. Data on historical milk intake and use of antacids and calcium supplements were also collected as part of the dietary section. Data were also collected on tobacco use, physical activity, reproductive health, medication use, and family history of osteoporosis.

Functional health status in the elderly

The functional health status component was designed to ascertain the prevalence of disability and limitations in function among the elderly. This component addressed three major areas: cognitive, physical, and social function.

Cognitive and physical function were assessed in the MEC and home examination for persons 60 years of age and over. Cognitive assessment consisted of a short paragraph given as an immediate and delayed recall task as part of the MEC Adult Questionnaire or the home examination. Physical function was assessed with a short battery of physical performance tests chosen to test different aspects of physical function important in everyday life. The measures included: range of motion of the shoulder, timed task of hand function (using a key to open a lock), rising out of a chair without the use of arms and timed rising five times from a chair in similar fashion, mobility of the hip and knee, timed task of balance (tandem stand), and timed walk with counting of steps on an 8-foot course.

Cognitive function among persons 60 years of age and over was assessed in the Household Adult Questionnaire through administration of a modified version of the Mini-Mental State Examination (46). The questions included counting backward from 20 by 3's and immediate and delayed recall of 3 items. In addition, all persons 17 years of age and over were assessed for orientation to location and date in the Household Adult Questionnaire.

For persons aged 60 years and over, the Household Adult Questionnaire contained standard questionnaire items on physical function derived from the NHANES I Epidemiologic Followup Study and the Supplement on Aging to the 1984 National Health Interview Survey. These items included questions on performance of activities of daily living and need for help and several questions directed to instrumental activities of daily living and need for help. Questions directed toward higher level function such as walking distances and climbing stairs were also included.

For adults aged 17 years and over, the Household Adult Questionnaire contained questions on social support. The questions included information on contact with friends and family members, attendance at organized religious activities, and involvement in other types of organizations.

Allergy

The primary element of the allergy component consisted of assessment of skin-test reactivity to standardized allergens. Related information includes data collected in the respiratory disease component.

Skin-prick tests were administered in the MEC to all examinees 6–19 years of age and to a random half-sample of examinees 20–59 years of age who were assigned to receive the allergy tests if their identification number ended in an even digit. Immediate hypersensitivity to any of

10 licensed commercially available allergens (mite, cat, short ragweed, perennial rye, alternaria, Bermuda grass, cockroach, Russian thistle, white oak, peanut) was determined. Histamine phosphate was used as a positive control and 50-percent glycerol saline was used as a negative control. The skin reactions were read 15–20 minutes after the skin was punctured and the allergens applied. Both the length and width of the wheal and flare were measured.

The Household Adult Questionnaire, administered to adults aged 17 years and over, included an extensive series of questions on respiratory symptoms related to allergies. The questions were designed to obtain information on trigger factors, severity, medication use, and hospitalization. An additional question ascertained previous diagnosis of asthma. The Household Youth Questionnaire included a similar set of questions for children aged 2 months–16 years.

Immunization and infectious diseases

Almost all infectious agents—bacteria, viruses, and parasites—elicit long-lasting and detectable immunity in the host. Therefore, NHANES III provides an important opportunity to study the seroepidemiology of the following infectious diseases: hepatitis A, B, C, and delta, herpes simplex I and II, human immunodeficiency virus (HIV), varicella, hantavirus, and Toxoplasma gondii. In addition, antibodies to the following microbial agents have been determined to assess the level of protective antibody in the population: tetanus, diphtheria, and rubella. Finally, antibody to Cryptosporidia parvum will be determined in sample persons from selected communities to assess exposure to this water-borne pathogen based on water source.

Serologic tests for antibodies will provide national estimates of exposure to hepatitis A, B, C, delta, and E and will assist in validating surveys that are more localized or that involve samples with potential sources of bias not found in NHANES. Because hepatitis A, B, and delta were performed on NHANES II (1976–80) sera, trends over time in the prevalence of infection can be determined (47). Hepatitis C virus is the name assigned to a newly detected virus that is thought to be the primary cause of transfusion-associated non-A, non-B hepatitis in the United States (48, 49). Testing of the NHANES III sera provides the unique opportunity to produce a baseline measure of the extent of infection in the U.S. population by this agent. The presence of specific antibodies directed against herpes simplex I and II will also be determined by serology. The population prevalence estimate will be used as a comparison for validating reporting systems involving patient-based and other smaller studies. NHANES II surplus sera were also previously tested for antibodies to these viral agents (50). Continuation of herpes serologic testing in NHANES III will produce trend data that will help to delineate the extent of a possible herpes epidemic. Other information related to sexual behavior and history of genital herpes was collected in the MEC Youth and MEC Adult Questionnaires.

Human immunodeficiency virus (HIV) testing was performed on all sample people over the age of 18 years using an anonymous protocol. Serum collected for the many other laboratory tests was separated into a vial that had been randomly numbered and not linked to the sample person's identification number. The only demographic information attached to the HIV sample was: age in 20-year groups, sex, race or ethnic group, and sampling location. In Phase 2 of the survey, a basic sampling weight, an education variable, and the results of the urine drug testing were also linked to the HIV result. Sample people were notified during the informed consent process that blood samples would be tested for HIV. As with any other component of the survey, the sample person had the right to refuse the test. The anonymous testing procedure was chosen for the HIV antibody testing to provide the maximum safeguard of the sample person's confidentiality. Anonymous testing was considered the only feasible method to provide unbiased estimates of seroprevalence of HIV antibody. The HIV prevalence estimate on a representative sample of the U.S. population will contribute further to the knowledge of the epidemiology of the disease previously obtained from select populations in the Center for Disease Control and Prevention's family of surveys (51, 52) and the distribution of reported cases.

A candidate vaccine for varicella has been developed and is currently undergoing final clinical trials prior to anticipated application for licensure for use in the United States. The seroprevalence and risk factors for varicella infection need to be established to better plan for wide use of this vaccine. NHANES III data will be used to target at-risk populations in the United States.

Because of the outbreak of adult respiratory disease syndrome caused by a newly described hantavirus during the summer of 1993, sera from NHANES III specimens were tested to determine the geographical distribution and prevalence of viruses in this family. These data will help quantify the extent of infection in the United States with these viruses to better assess the potential for additional cases of this often-fatal illness. The results of the testing will also immediately affect CDC educational efforts and surveillance activities directed against this virus.

Because congenital toxoplasmosis often leads to mental retardation, visual impairment, deafness, or death in an infected infant, prevention of maternal infection is critical. To look at the cost-benefit relationship of a screening program for women to prevent this infection, an accurate estimate of the prevalence of infection in the United States must be made. Determination of risk factors for women who become infected with T. gondii will help in targeting prevention strategies. The use of NHANES III serologic specimens to assess prevalence is essential to develop recommendations for prevention of congenital toxoplasmosis and to address the risk of exposure to acquired immunodeficiency syndrome (AIDS) patients.

The following serologic tests were performed to determine the level of protective antibody elicited by the respective vaccines. This is an important component of the U.S. immunization initiative. A tetanus antibody titer was determined to indicate the level of protection for all examinees 4 years of age and over. Children aged 2 months–16 years (or the parent or guardian) were asked if the children had ever had a diphtheria-pertussis- tetanus (DPT) shot and if so, when the last shot was given. In addition, diphtheria antitoxin levels were determined in sera specimens because of evidence that this component of the DPT vaccine may elicit a weaker immune response and provide reduced levels of protection against this bacterial toxin. Because of recent outbreaks of measles and rubella, inclusion of a serologic test for rubella antibody using NHANES III specimens will provide information on populations at risk for these viruses.

Hearing

The principal elements in the hearing component were the measurements of pure tone air conduction audiometric thresholds and tympanic compliance in children. These examinations, pure tone audiometry and tympanometry, were conducted in a soundproof room in the MEC for examinees aged 6–19 years. Pure tone air conduction audiometry thresholds were obtained in both ears at 500, 1000, 2000, 3000, 4000, 6000, and 8000 hz. A screening questionnaire administered before the examination provided data on recent noise exposure and use of headphones. Because pure tone screening by itself may not be sensitive enough to detect middle ear disease, tympanometry was conducted to provide an estimate of tympanic membrane compliance. The Household Adult Questionnaire, administered to adults aged 17 years and over, collected information on hearing status and use of hearing aids.

The Household Youth Questionnaire included questions on frequency and treatment of ear infections, hearing status, and hearing aid use for children aged 2 months–16 years.

Lead exposure

The lead exposure component was designed to assess environmental lead exposure through measurement of blood lead levels. Blood lead levels were determined on examinees 1 year of age and over on specimens collected by venipuncture during the MEC or home examination. Analysis was performed by graphite furnace atomic absorption spectrophotometry. Erythrocyte protoporphyrin, a screening test only sensitive to high lead levels, was also measured.

The Household Youth Questionnaire included questions on history of testing and treatment for lead poisoning for children aged 2 months–16 years. Information on the age of the housing structure was also collected in the Family Questionnaire.

Mental health and neurobehavioral function

The primary elements of the mental health and neurobehavioral function component were conducted in the MEC and included assessment of depression and mania, cognitive function, and functioning of the central nervous system. Supplemental data were collected in the household interview.

The mental health and neurobehavioral function component of NHANES III included the depression and mania subsections from the Diagnostic Interview Schedule (DIS), developed by the National Institute of Mental Health (NIMH). Sections of the DIS have also been used in the Hispanic HANES and in several community studies (53–55). Trained interviewers administered the NHANES III DIS questions in the MEC, using automated data entry, as part of the MEC Youth Questionnaire for examinees 15–16 years of age and as part of the MEC Adult

II-17

Questionnaire for examinees 17–39 years of age. The data collected from the DIS permit diagnoses based on the third edition of the Diagnostic and Statistical Manual of Mental Disorders (DSM-III)(56).

Intellectual function and academic performance were assessed for children aged 6–16 years with standardized cognitive tests. The examination included the block design and digit-span subtests from the Wechsler Intelligence Scale for Children, Revised (WISC-R) (57) and the reading and arithmetic sections from the Wide Range Achievement Test, Revised (WRAT-R) (58).

Central nervous system function was assessed with a set of simple, nonverbal performance tests designed to be minimally influenced by differences in language or education. The tests were administered to a random half-sample of all adults 20–59 years of age, who were assigned to receive these tests if their identification number ended in an odd digit. The examination was composed of three tests—simple reaction time, serial digit learning, and symbol digit substitution—selected from the larger battery of Neurobehavioral Evaluation System (NES) tests (59). Factors that might have affected performance such as motivation, use of drugs, alcohol, or caffeine, and the temperature, humidity, and air flow in the testing booth were recorded in a brief pre- and post-test questionnaire.

The Household Youth Questionnaire, administered to children aged 2 months–16 years, included questions on attendance to special classes in school as a result of impairment and diagnosis of mental retardation. Data were also collected on visits to a psychiatrist, psychologist, or psychoanalyst for children 4–16 years of age and on school attendance and relationships with friends for those 5–16 years of age. The Household Youth Questionnaire also included a series of questions on motor and social development for children aged 2 months–3 years. The questions were modeled after the Denver Developmental Screening Test (60) and a similar component used in the Child Health Supplement to the 1981 National Health Interview Survey. Related information includes occupational history and the cognitive, physical, and social function data collected in the functional health status of the elderly component.

Oral health

The main element of the oral health component was an oral examination conducted in the MEC. Methods used in this component were designed to be consistent with previous health examination surveys conducted by NCHS and with previous national surveys of oral health conducted by the National Institute for Dental Research (NIDR). Related information was also collected on selected risk factors such as diet, the use of smokeless tobacco, and the use of fluoride supplements.

During the MEC examination, the dentist performed oral examinations on all examinees 12 months of age and over. Oral soft tissue lesions were assessed for examinees aged 2 years and over. The assessment involved visual observation of the oral mucosa and laboratory assessment of an oral mucosal smear for the presence of hyphae of candida albicans. A dental caries examination included an evaluation of coronal caries for those aged 2 years and over, root surface caries for examinees 18 years and over, and baby-bottle tooth decay among children aged 12–23 months. Examinees were questioned about history of injury to front teeth and then were examined for evidence of traumatic injury to the four upper and four lower permanent incisors.

Occlusal characteristics were assessed in examinees aged 8–50 years and included measurement of the alignment of teeth and assessment of posterior crossbite, overjet, overbite, and maxillary diastema. A periodontal examination was performed on two randomly selected quadrants of the mouth for examinees 13 years of age and over. Restorations and tooth conditions for those 18–74 years were also evaluated.

The Household Adult Questionnaire, administered to adults 17 years of age and over, included questions on utilization of dental health services and information needed to interpret the oral examination findings, such as history of cold sores and receipt of orthodontic treatment. The Household Youth Questionnaire included similar questions for children aged 2–16 years, as well as infant feeding practices contributing to baby bottle caries.

Risk factors and health behaviors

Risk factors and health behaviors associated with many chronic diseases and conditions were evaluated in NHANES III both in the household interview and during the MEC examination. The five primary behaviors assessed in the survey were alcohol use, tobacco use, drug use, physical activity, and sexual experience. The component on drug use is described in the special studies topic of this section.

Alcohol use

The MEC Youth and MEC Adult Questionnaires included questions on alcohol use for all examinees 12 years of age and over. The questions were designed to identify nondrinkers, very light drinkers, and former heavy drinkers; to ascertain quantity and frequency of use for quantifying alcohol intake; and to determine the frequency of heavy drinking occasions. Data on any alcohol intake during the previous day were also recorded for all examinees as part of the 24-hour dietary recall. The section on "Nutritional health assessment" of this report also has some information on alcohol. Standard liver function tests were performed. The Household Adult Questionnaire, administered to adults 17 years of age and over, included questions on the frequency of consumption of beer, wine, and liquor as part of the food frequency section.

Tobacco use and exposure

To encourage honest reporting of tobacco use by youths aged 8–16 years, information on use of cigarettes and smokeless tobacco (snuff or chewing tobacco) was collected in the privacy of the MEC as part of the MEC Youth Questionnaire. Data were collected on age of initiation, frequency, duration, and amount of tobacco consumed. Recent use of tobacco or nicotine gum within the past 5 days, for evaluation of laboratory results, was also assessed in the MEC Youth and MEC Adult Questionnaires and the home examination for those aged 8 years and over.

The Household Adult Questionnaire, administered to adults 17 years of age and over, included questions on the use of cigarettes, cigars, pipes, and smokeless tobacco (snuff or chewing tobacco). Data were collected on age of initiation, frequency, duration, and amount of tobacco consumed and on exposure to tobacco smoke at work. Data on passive smoke exposure were collected in the Family Questionnaire. Family members who smoked cigarettes in the home were identified and the amount smoked per day was estimated. The Household Youth Questionnaire included questions on history of maternal smoking during pregnancy for children aged 2 months–11 years.

A biochemical determination of tobacco exposure was used to assess both passive smoking and tobacco use through measurement of blood cotinine levels from specimens obtained by venipuncture in the MEC from examinees aged 4 years and over. Cotinine is a metabolite of nicotine and is thus an indicator of primary or secondary exposure to tobacco. Cotinine was detected using an isotope dilution, liquid chromatography, tandem mass spectrometry method developed by the National Center for Environmental Health, CDC, which conducted the analyses. This was a newly developed method designed to detect levels as low as 0.030 nanograms per milliliter. Related information includes data collected in the respiratory disease component and identification of oral soft tissue lesions in the oral health component.

Physical activity

For children 8–16 years of age, data on frequency of exercise and physical activity were collected
during the MEC interview. The Household Adult Questionnaire, administered to adults aged 17 years and over, contained questions on leisure-time physical activity adapted from the1985 National Health Interview Survey and included information on types of activity, frequency, and assessment of level of activity compared with others. Participants were also asked to compare current levels of physical activity with those of the past year and 10 years ago. Related information includes data collected in the functional health status of the elderly component.

Sexual experience

Questions on sexual experience were included in the MEC Youth and MEC Adult Questionnaires for examinees aged 15–59 years. Information on age at first sexual intercourse, total number of partners, and number of partners in the past year was collected for those 17–59 years of age. Males 17–59 years of age were asked about the numbers of male and female partners. Age at first sexual intercourse was obtained from youths aged 15–16 years. Related information includes data collected in the immunization and infectious disease and reproductive health components.

Special studies

Four special studies requiring an additional collection of blood or urine during the MEC examination were carried out in conjunction with NHANES III. Planned and sponsored with other agencies, their unique status was warranted either by the confidential or experimental design of the research. The two highly sensitive studies, HIV testing and drug testing, were conducted using a rigorous protocol that maximized anonymity and confidentiality. The HIV testing is described in the immunization and infectious diseases section. The results from these analyses can only be linked to a limited set of demographic and medical information collected in the survey. The priority toxicant range study and the establishment of a deoxyribonucleic acid (DNA) storage bank for genetic research were both designed, in part, to explore new and experimental laboratory techniques. Also, a portion of the sera was placed in a bank for unanticipated future research projects.

Drug use

All examinees aged 12 years and over were questioned in the MEC Adult and Youth Questionnaires about lifetime and past-month use of marijuana and cocaine. In Phase 2 of NHANES III (1991–94), anonymous urine testing was included in the MEC examination in order to detect the presence of marijuana, cocaine, phencyclidine (PCP), opiates (morphine and codeine), and stimulants (amphetamine and methamphetamine) among examinees 18–59 years of age. Urine specimens were randomly numbered so they could not be linked with the examinee identification numbers. Limited demographic data including age (in 20-year categories), sex, race or ethnicity, sampling location, and educational level were included with the random numbers on protected data files. The identical random numbers and the associated demographic variables were assigned to the HIV serum, so that the association between drug use and HIV status could be examined.

Specimens were screened using an enzyme multiplied immunoassay technique with cutoff concentrations lower than those generally used in drug screening. Positive specimens were confirmed and then quantified using gas chromatography mass spectrometry. Urine analyses for drug screening were performed in a National Institute of Drug Abuse (NIDA) certified laboratory according to NIDA guidelines.

Priority toxicant reference range study

The purpose of the priority toxicant reference range study was to assess the levels of common pesticides and volatile organic compounds (VOC's) in a large sample of the U.S. population and to evaluate laboratory analytic methods in the process. Two groups of organic compounds were measured in the priority toxicant study: selected pesticides and their metabolites at the low parts-per-billion levels in urine and VOC's at the low parts-per-trillion levels in whole blood (see appendix table VII). The Division of Environmental Health Laboratory Sciences, National Center for Environmental Health, CDC, conducted the Priority Toxicant Reference Range Study on approximately 3,600 persons aged 20–59 years examined in NHANES III. Participants volunteered to complete a brief chemical exposure questionnaire and to provide an additional 20 ml of blood and 40 ml of urine. No formal sampling procedures were instituted; 45 volunteers participated at each survey location. A $10 remuneration was awarded for participation. Demographic and medical information obtained from NHANES III can be linked to the resulting laboratory measurements.

Serum bank and DNA specimen bank

NHANES III provided an opportunity to establish two nationally representative specimen banks, a serum specimen bank and a DNA bank of preserved, viable cells. Serum specimens are stored at -70 °C or less and will be used for unanticipated future research projects.

For the DNA analyses, new molecular genetic techniques make it possible to examine substantial portions of the DNA sequence and its variation in the population using small samples of nucleated cells obtained by venipuncture. The development of transformation and immortalization procedures to maintain active cultures of cells means that small samples collected from a large population can be maintained and amplified to provide specimens for future studies. It is anticipated that this endeavor will help establish a new era of health research that integrates genetics and environmental factors in the understanding of human disease.

During the MEC examination, a 6-cm^3 specimen of venous blood was collected in a vacutainer tube containing a Ficoll heavy-density layer overlaid with a thixotropic gel followed by ACD anticoagulant from examinees 12 years of age and over. The specimen was then prepared by the National Center for Environmental Health following one of two methods. Either the nucleated cells were separated from the blood sample and then separated in several aliquots or the cells were separated from the blood sample and virally transformed to yield an immortalized culture. In both instances, multiple aliquots from each subject were frozen, following a controlled freezing procedure. The frozen aliquots are maintained in liquid nitrogen.

APPENDIX III

NHANES III Nutritional Status Assessment

(Note: The material in this Appendix is taken verbatim from the NCHS source document. A list of the references cited in the original NCHS document has not been included in this Appendix. The reader is referred to the source document for the full citations.)

(Source: NCHS, 1994b, pp. 12-17.)

NUTRITIONAL STATUS ASSESSMENT

Nutrition data from the National Health and Nutrition Examination Survey (NHANES) are vital to nutrition monitoring and public health. As the cornerstone of the "nutrition and related health measurement" component of the Federal Government's National Nutrition Monitoring and Related Research Program (NNMRRP) (61), NHANES nutrition data are used in a variety of settings to enhance the health and nutritional status of the Nation. NHANES III data will be used to track progress toward the Nation's health and nutrition objectives (62,63,16) for diet, serum cholesterol, hypertension, iron deficiency anemia, overweight, and infant feeding practices. Additionally, NHANES provides reference data for nutritional biochemistries (64–72), anthropometric measures (73–76,8), and nutrient intakes (77–78); and provides information for policymakers to set nutrition policy (16,62,79–82) and research agendas (79,83,84). NHANES III was also designed to demonstrate relationships between diet and health. The nutritional assessments were designed to complement and link to NHANES III health components such as cardiovascular disease, diabetes, hypertension, osteoporosis, and dental caries to maximize data utility. A longitudinal design was added to the traditional NHANES cross-sectional design and studies of the relationship between present diet and future disease will be possible.

Food and nutrient consumption

Dietary factors are associated with 5 of the 10 leading causes of death and are associated with other conditions such as obesity (16). Deficiencies of nutrients and minerals, such as iron and some vitamins, remain a problem in selected population subgroups. Inadequate food intake and undernutrition are problems in high-risk subgroups such as low-income populations. Overconsumption of food components such as fat, cholesterol, and salt and underconsumption of fruits, vegetables, and complex carbohydrates are significant problems in the general population. Measurement of nutrient intake is important in evaluating food fortification, nutrition education, and intervention programs aimed at improving the population's dietary intake. Measurement of foods as they contribute to nutrient intake and as they comprise dietary patterns are important for evaluating and developing dietary guidance (81). Recognizing the importance of measuring both nutrient intake and food intake to meet current nutrition monitoring data needs, the NHANES III dietary component was developed to estimate total nutrient intake, nutrient intake from foods, intake of specific foods, and problems and factors related to insufficient food and nutrient intake.

Vitamin and mineral supplement data will be used by NCHS and the Food and Drug Administration (FDA) to determine the prevalence of very low and very high total nutrient intake levels in the population and for assessing the contribution of supplements to total nutrient intake and nutritional status (83). Total nutrient intake is also important for evaluating diet-health relationships such as the association between total calcium intake, blood pressure, and hypertension risk (84), and total calcium intake and bone density (85–86).

Alcohol intake

Alcohol problems and associated health risks are prevalent problems in adolescents and adults (16). Excessive alcohol intake is associated with cirrhosis of the liver as well as accidents and suicides (16). Moderate amounts of alcohol have been related to both increased risk of certain cancers and decreased risk of coronary heart disease (87). Information on alcohol was collected in NHANES III to quantify the contribution of alcohol to total caloric intake for population reference data, to assess the proportion of the population who typically consume larger amounts of alcohol than recommended in the Dietary Guidelines for Americans (81), and to investigate the relationship between alcohol intake and health outcomes (87,15).

Food program participation and food security

In the 1980's there were several reports that indicated that hunger was a serious problem in the United States on a national level and for certain subgroups of the population (88–93). However, accurately estimating the prevalence and severity of hunger is complex and historically has been controversial. In 1987, the University of California at Berkeley sponsored a workshop to bring together hunger researchers working at the local, State, and national levels. The workshop concluded that "of all the relevant Federal surveys, NHANES is probably the best equipped to look at the interrelationships between diet, food shortages, and health indicators" (94).

In addition to questions for families and individuals about having enough food or money to buy food, data were collected in NHANES III about the use of food stamps, participation in the Special Supplemental Food Program for Women, Infants, and Children (WIC), school breakfast and school lunch programs, and elderly feeding programs. Assessment of the dietary status of participants of such programs is important in aiding the study of Federal food programs and their effect on the dietary intake of low-income and high-risk subgroups.

NHANES III will enable researchers to link food security and program participation with other nutrition and health indicators, including cognitive function. This is especially important for children. It has been documented that hungry children can be irritable, apathetic, or lethargic, which can interfere with learning (95). The National Education Goals were established in 1990, the first of which states that by the year 2000, "all children in America will start school ready to learn" (96). Having adequate food is a large part of this.

Vitamin and mineral status

Biochemical and hematological indicators of nutritional status are an essential part of the NHANES III nutrition component. Blood assessments have been included in past NHANES to determine the prevalence of compromised vitamin and mineral status at both the high and low ends of the population distribution (64–72); and the prevalence of nutrition-related risk factors, such as elevated serum cholesterol (10,11,97,98) or serum albumin (68).

Assessing fat-soluble vitamin status is of interest because of the widespread use of vitamin and mineral supplements in this country, coupled with the toxic potential of vitamin A (87) and the recent development of fat substitutes in food, which may influence fat-soluble vitamin absorption (87). In addition, serum levels of antioxidants, including alpha-tocopherol, carotenoids, selenium, and vitamin C, are of interest because of their possible role in reducing the risk of some cancers and heart disease (87). Finally, serum assays for the heavy metals lead and cadmium were included to assess toxicities of these contaminants and to correlate them with other health measures.

History of the use of certain drugs was ascertained because such use may be related to specific diseases. For example, long-term use of antacids containing calcium may be related to bone densitometry or blood pressure. In addition, chronic use of aspirin could affect risk of heart disease, stroke, or gallstones. This information will be used to assess the potential interaction of nutritional status and medications.

Iron-deficiency anemia

Iron deficiency has been described as the most common single nutritional deficiency in the developed and developing countries (64,68,72,99,100). Iron deficiency continues to be a special concern for children and women in poverty and women of childbearing age. NHANES II showed that 9 percent of children 1–2 years of age, 4 percent of children 3–4 years of age, and 5 percent of women aged 20–44 years had iron-deficiency anemia (16,68,72). The prevalence in low income women and children was even higher. Because iron depletion develops gradually (72,100), a battery of iron-status indicators was included in NHANES III to assess all stages of iron deficiency. Most of these indicators have also been included in previous NHANES, so it will be possible to examine secular trends.

Folate deficiency

There is some evidence that low serum folate levels in pregnant women are associated with neural tube defects in their infants (101,102). The Centers for Disease Control and Prevention (CDC), Food and Drug Administration, and other Public Health Service agencies are considering food fortification changes to increase folate intake in the target population, i.e., women of childbearing age (103). Assessment of anemia resulting from folate deficiency will be possible because of the availability of serum and red cell folate, dietary folate, and supplement-usage data in NHANES III. Because high intakes of folate can mask vitamin B12 deficiency, it is also important to have a measure of vitamin B12 status. An assessment of this status was added to Phase 2 in NHANES III to estimate the prevalence of vitamin B12 deficiency in the population and to establish a baseline for evaluating future changes in folate food fortification policy.

Infant and child nutrition

Infants and children are particularly vulnerable to poor nutrition. Childhood and adolescence are important periods for establishing nutrition and health habits for later life. Whether or not an infant is breastfed, the type of milk or infant formula an infant is fed, and the types of solid foods first introduced are all critical infant feeding practices. Adequate dietary intake during infancy and childhood is necessary for proper growth and development and the prevention of future health problems. Of particular concern at this early age are iron deficiency, poor dietary habits, breastfeeding, and inadequate intake in high-risk populations (95). Also, overconsumption of certain foods is related to the development of obesity and dental caries in children.

Growth

Anthropometric measurements have been included in the National Health Examination Surveys since the first National Health Examination Survey (NHES I) was conducted in 1960–62 (1,104). These measurements were the basis for the NCHS growth charts, which were constructed with data from the earlier health examination surveys. The charts are used nationally in hospitals, health departments, and physicians' offices and have been adopted for international use by the World Health Organization (105,106). The production of these original growth charts, however, was affected by some inherent limitations. Because data were not available in previous NCHS surveys for the very youngest age group (age under 1 year), the data were supplemented with data from the Fels Research Institute (8). This resulted in growth curves for recumbent length (for children from birth through 3 years of age) based on Fels data and for stature (for children aged 2–18 years) based on NCHS data. Because the median statures for the Fels data were greater than the median statures in the NCHS data, there was a disjuncture in the curves for children between 24 and 36 months of age (107). NHANES III was specifically designed to resolve both of these limitations; children 2 months of age and over were included in the survey (108), and more sophisticated curve-smoothing techniques that have evolved since the first NCHS growth charts will be used.

Overweight and obesity

Overweight and obesity are current public health issues and prevalent risk factors for chronic disease. NHANES III anthropometric data will be used to estimate the prevalence of overweight and severe overweight in the United States for various age, race or ethnicity, and gender subgroups (16,74). NHANES II data showed that 26 percent of adults were overweight (16). Assessment of body fat distribution has been shown to be related to chronic disease development (87). Body measurement data indicative of overweight or obesity will be used as control or explanatory variables in epidemiological analyses of many other examination items, including blood pressure, glucose intolerance, gallbladder ultrasound, and a battery of other indicators for cardiovascular disease.

Anthropometric measures can be utilized in many ways; for example, to estimate body composition, to develop various reference standards, to establish baseline data for future longitudinal studies, to monitor trends over time in the population, and to evaluate risks for adverse health outcomes (109).

Diet-health relationships

With the growing understanding of the role of nutrition in health promotion and disease prevention, nutritional status assessment has assumed greater prominence and has been integrally linked with other aspects of NHANES III. As the Surgeon General remarked upon the release of The Surgeon General's Report on Nutrition and Health (15), for the majority of adults who don't smoke and don't drink excessively, what they eat is the most significant controllable risk factor affecting their long-term health. The NHANES III has been designed to capture as many nutrition risk factors as feasible related to the major chronic diseases affecting Americans, while continuing to provide a comprehensive assessment of the population's nutritional status for nutrition monitoring purposes.

The dietary information will be useful for studying the relationship between dietary habits and health. For example, sodium-intake data from the dietary interview, more specific than in past NHANES, can be linked with blood pressure data, saturated fat can be linked to blood cholesterol, and intake of antioxidants such as vitamins A, C, E, and carotenoids can be joined with followup information on cancer and heart disease (15). Past NHANES data have been used to relate the number of meals and snacks eaten to dental caries (110); and information on the number of meals eaten away from home can be used to plan and evaluate nutrition education programs targeting overweight and obese clients.

Osteoporosis and calcium intake

Osteoporosis is a debilitating disease of reduced bone mass that causes fractures of the vertebrae, hip, forearm, and other bones. Intake of calcium, phosphorus, vitamin D, protein, and alcohol, as well as a sedentary lifestyle, may all be related to the development of osteoporosis (111). NHANES III measures intake of these nutrients, including total calcium and frequency of consumption of calcium-rich foods. In addition, a question on historical intake of milk was included in the household interview to investigate the relationship between past calcium intake and current bone densitometry results. Interest in past consumption of dairy foods has been raised by findings suggesting that the level of calcium intake by young adults may be related to peak bone mass (85,86).

Nutritional status methods

The nutritional assessment component of NHANES III was designed to include several data sources (dietary intake interviews, nutrition-related interviews, anthropometric data, hematological and nutritional biochemistries, and nutrition-related clinical assessments) in order to provide a comprehensive assessment of nutritional status (112).

Methodologies for the nutritional assessment were developed with input from experts and data users from government agencies, academic research institutions, and industry. In 1986, an NHANES III Nutrition Methodology Working Group was established. In addition to NCHS planning staff, it included Federal staff with specific expertise in the topics under discussion and/or who were primary data users with a nutrition policy need for the data. The Nutrition Methodology Working Group reviewed the literature and discussed survey methods, operational issues, and specific details that needed to be determined for the NHANES III nutrition component. Planning sessions included discussion of the following topics:

• General issues. Household versus mobile examination center (MEC) administration of the dietary interview; automated data collection; nutrition monitoring and comparability to other national surveys, primarily the food consumption surveys conducted by the U.S. Department of Agriculture (USDA).

• 24-hour dietary recall method. Automated versus manual data collection; number of days of observation; location of interview; number of interviews per individual; adults versus children in the household.

• Food frequency questionnaire (FFQ). Review of FFQ's used in other surveys, including past NHANES and the 1987 National Health Interview Survey; appropriate uses of FFQ data.

• Longitudinal study issues relative to nutrition.

• Children's issues. Proxy rules; use of food models; data retrieval for day care and school lunch.

• Dietary questions. Interview information needed on food security (hunger); water intake; dietary practices.

• Vitamin and mineral supplement usage. Level of detail required; method of data collection.

• Anthropometry. Measurements; bioelectrical impedance; supplemental interview questions (e.g., self-assessment of overweight).

Based on the study objectives, consideration of outside input, and the Nutrition Methodology Working Group discussions, a comprehensive nutrition proposal was developed by NCHS staff. The proposal was reviewed by NHANES III Research Consortium members and served as the basis for planning the nutrition component.

Dietary methodology

Prior NHANES conducted between 1971 and 1984 included 24-hour dietary recall and food frequency components as parts of the dietary interview (77,113). On March 16–18, 1986, NCHS sponsored the Dietary Methodology Workshop to review dietary methodologies and obtain recommendations for selection of methods for NHANES III (114). Experts in the fields of dietary survey methodology, epidemiology, nutrition, public health, and biostatistics presented papers that addressed statistical issues unique to the interpretation and use of dietary survey data, selection of dietary methods appropriate for nutrition monitoring activities, and approaches useful for assessing the relationship of diet to energy balance and three diet-related chronic diseases (cancer, cardiovascular disease, and osteoporosis) (114).

The overall workshop recommendation, based on the major aims of the NHANES III nutrition component, was that NCHS should continue to use the 24-hour recall as the principal methodology to provide detailed quantitative food and nutrient intake data for the U.S. population. Use of a food frequency was recommended to supplement data from the 24-hour recall and to provide typical or qualitative data for ranking persons by intake of specific foods and food groups.

Twenty-four-hour dietary recall

The 24-hour recall was collected through an automated interview using the Dietary Data Collection (DDC) system (appendix I). All NHANES III examinees, approximately 30,000 total, were asked to complete a 24-hour dietary recall during their MEC visit. In addition, about 5 percent of all adult examinees received a second replicate MEC examination that included a 24-hour dietary recall; replicate data will be used to estimate within- and between-person variances for estimating nutrient intake distributions. NHANES III examinations were conducted on all days of the week with the objective of conducting approximately 15 percent of the 24-hour recalls on each day of the week.

NHANES III, Phase 1 examinees 50 years of age and over (approximately 3,500 persons) who completed a 24-hour recall interview in the MEC were eligible to participate in a special dietary study of older persons—the Supplemental Nutrition Survey of Older Americans (SNSOA) (115,116). The SNSOA was funded through an interagency agreement with the National Institute on Aging at the NIH. The objective of the study was to obtain two independent replicate 24-hour recalls, administered by trained telephone interviewers, using the DDC system. Replicate 24-hour recall data will be used to estimate usual intakes of older persons, to adjust nutrient intake estimates, and to explore methodologic issues (116).

The SNSOA telephone methodology was pretested in two pilot studies. SNSOA subjects were recontacted by telephone interviewers approximately 8 and 16 months after their MEC examination. Most of the telephone interviews were unscheduled and subjects were not compensated for their participation in the SNSOA. Appendix table IX indicates the administration of the 24-hour dietary recall and the FFQ in NHANES III by age of the sample person, respondent (self and/or proxy), place of interview (sample person's home or MEC), and interview type (nondietary, dietary, and telephone).

Food frequency

In a major innovation for the NHANES, a FFQ was incorporated into the household interview to provide general qualitative dietary information for individuals aged 17 years and over. The FFQ used a 1-month reference period and was not quantitative, i.e., did not collect portion sizes. It was not designed to produce population nutrient intake estimates, and use of food frequency data for this purpose is not appropriate (109,117–119).

The FFQ food list was developed to be comparable to food lists used in past NHANES for trend assessment but was expanded to capture more detailed intake of foods containing specific nutrients of interest. Foods containing nutrients related to risk for cancer, cardiovascular disease, and osteoporosis (87), such as vitamins A and C, caffeine, and calcium, respectively, were added to a general food list. In addition, the instrument was modified to be appropriate for use with the population subgroups sampled in NHANES III by including foods high in these nutrients that were reported by white and black persons in NHANES II and by Mexican-Americans in Hispanic HANES.

Because the FFQ was collected during the household interview, information on food intake is available for all interviewed persons and can also be linked with reported health conditions. Collection of the FFQ in the household for all interviewed persons will also allow assessment of potential nonresponse to the 24-hour recall, which was collected in the MEC for interviewed and examined persons. Another important use of the food frequency data is to provide baseline dietary data for followup analysis. Because all NHANES III sample persons are followed for mortality, a larger sample of interviewed persons with dietary intake information is available for followup analysis.

To complement the osteoporosis component, adults were asked to report their milk consumption during five age periods: 5–12 years, 13–17 years, 18–35 years, 36–65 years, and 65 years of age and over. Responses were recorded as "more than once per day," "once per day," "less than once per day, but more than once per week," "once per week," "less than once per week," or "never." Although several researchers have found that the recall of past diet was strongly influenced by present dietary habits (120–124) and that it is difficult to quantify the amount of calcium consumed during periods of peak bone growth using retrospective dietary data, most people can probably retrospectively report whether or not they consumed milk products during these time periods in a qualitative sense.

Nutrition-related interview

A complete picture of dietary intake is not possible with a single 24-hour recall and food frequency. Therefore, additional interview questions were asked about water intake, usage of vitamin and mineral supplements, meal and snack patterns, infant feeding practices, alcohol intake, and food sufficiency. Appendix table X shows the nutrition-related interview information collected in NHANES III by age of individual.

Questions related to periodic or chronic food shortages were asked for both families and individuals to study the impact of food insecurity on dietary intake, nutritional status, and health (88). At the family level, questions were asked about the number of days per month on which there was no food or money to buy food and the reasons for the problem. The questions for individuals, modeled after those developed and used in the Community Childhood Hunger Identification Project (125), asked about the frequency of and reasons for skipping meals and going without food (88).

In addition to the 24-hour recall and food frequency, alcohol intake information was collected through additional questions about current and past alcohol consumption asked of respondents aged 12 years and over during a private interview in the MEC. When using and interpreting alcohol data from the various data collection methods used in NHANES III, it is important to note that alcohol intake estimates can vary between dietary methods because of method and reporting differences (126). To assess total nutrient intake, sources of nutrients such as discretionary salt, water, vitamin and mineral supplements, and nutrient-containing medicines were evaluated. The DDC system (i.e., 24-hour recall) was specifically designed to probe for fat and salt used in the preparation of foods, and additional questions about type and frequency of salt used at the table were asked. Usual daily water consumption and the amount of water consumed for the 24-hour recall period were collected. The source of the home water supply and the presence in the home of a water softening or conditioning system were assessed during the household interview. Serious consideration was given to the collection of a household drinking water sample, but it was decided that one casual water sample would not be representative of the usual content of household water for all seasons.

Information about current vitamin and mineral supplements and prescription and nonprescription medication usage for the month prior to the interview was collected during the household interview and for the 24-hour period prior to examination. If possible, the interviewer recorded brand and dosage directly from the supplement or prescription medication container label and asked about the frequency of usage.

Anthropometry

A core set of body measures has been included in all past NHANES; however, the necessity of certain measures and the availability of new equipment warranted the discontinuation of some measures and the addition of others. The current set of measures was selected from a public health perspective. Because of heightened awareness and the emergence of evidence of associations between fat distribution and health outcomes, the number of circumference measurements was expanded. Additionally, to be on the cutting edge of new technology amenable to the survey environment, bioelectrical impedance analysis (BIA) was included for those age groups for which stable prediction equations were expected to become available from empirical research (127).

The selection of both procedures and equipment was influenced by constraints inherent to the unique setting of this survey and by the need to ensure reasonable comparability with the past while collecting data to meet current needs. In order to include an optimal number of measures in a limited time frame, a considerable amount of planning and experimentation was devoted to modifying and refining applications of the equipment, the procedures, and the facility, including the automated data recording system. The final array of body measures was distilled to several sets that are variably administered, dependent upon the age of the sample persons. These measures are shown in appendix IV and may be categorized as weight, height, length, circumference, breadth, skinfold, and bioelectrical impedance.

As with all other components of this survey, the primary objective was to maximize validity and reliability. Because one major end product of the anthropometric component is to produce reference values, accuracy was emphasized through standardized training and a multifaceted quality control system. Related to this, reproducibility is also a paramount concern, not only within and between individual data collectors and trainers for NHANES III, but also to facilitate comparisons between the NHANES III and other surveys and studies. Specific consideration was given to selecting methods that incorporated, to the extent possible, objective procedures. For example, bony landmarks were selected to identify anatomical sites for placement of the instruments and proper positioning of the sample persons; marks were made on the measurement sites to locate midpoints and anchor the measuring devices; and where feasible, measures were taken directly on the skin. In general, the guidelines of the Anthropometric Standardization Reference Manual (128) were followed, although modifications were made for selected procedures. Documentation of complete details of the NHANES III anthropometric procedures will be disseminated in a separate publication.

Laboratory determinations

When selecting nutritional biochemistry and hematological indicators to include in NHANES III, first priority was given to scientific merit. An NCHS survey planning group was charged with developing a list of blood determinations for NHANES III, including priorities by age group. The planning group used recommendations from an ad hoc panel convened by the Life Sciences Research Office, Federation of American Societies for Experimental Biology, at the request of the FDA (100), as well as other important sources, such as the first report of the Joint Nutrition Monitoring Evaluation Committee (129) and The Surgeon General's Report on Nutrition and Health (15). Individual agencies and institutes within the NIH also developed specific proposals for biochemical and hematological measures to be included in NHANES III. For example, the National Heart, Lung, and Blood Institute developed and funded the lipid analysis for NHANES III (see the part "Health status assessment"). The scientific merit of each measure was evaluated in the context of the goals of the survey, i.e., which NHANES III health conditions and examination measures were available for linkage with the laboratory data.

If deemed to have sufficient scientific merit, the next criterion considered was feasibility of measuring the indicator in a national survey. This included whether the state-of-the-art analytic methodology currently accepted by the scientific community was practical for a large field survey lasting 6 years. Specimen size requirements and staff and monetary costs also had a bearing on feasibility (130). Laboratory protocols and analytical methods for several nutritional determinations were developed at the National Center for Environmental Health (CDC). A list of the nutritional biochemistry and hematological variables assayed in NHANES III is shown by age in appendix table IV. In previous NHANES, blood was collected from children by fingerstick. However, because of problems in performing a fingerstick without creating contamination or causing hemodilution by "milking," it was decided to collect blood from children aged 1 year and over in NHANES III by venipuncture only (130,131). Because a lesser amount of blood can be collected from children than from adults, it was not possible to assay the full battery of nutritional biochemistries in children. For young children, only the most critical nutritional biochemistries were assayed (appendix table IV).

One new indicator, red cell distribution width, was added because it may become abnormal earlier in the development of iron deficiency than other blood cell count indicators, such as hemoglobin or mean cell volume, but after the fall of iron stores (132). Many iron-status indicators are affected by inflammation as well as by iron deficiency (72). The ability to assess iron status in NHANES III has been enhanced by the addition of a biochemical measure of inflammation, C-reactive protein. The C-reactive protein measure, which will also be useful in the arthritis component, will aid determination of the prevalence of true iron deficiency without confounding by inflammatory conditions. This will be particularly useful when assessing iron status of older persons, in whom the prevalence of abnormal iron status indicators as a result of inflammation is high (133).

Serum and red blood cell folate were assessed on all examined persons 4 years of age and over. For Phase 2 of the survey (1991–94), assessment of homocysteine, methylmalonic acid, and vitamin B12 were added to provide population reference data on vitamin B12 status. This information will be critical to assessing the population's folate status and folate-vitamin B12 relationships.

NHANES III provides the most comprehensive assessment of fat-soluble vitamin status available from an NHANES. In addition to vitamins A and E, which have been measured in at least one previous NHANES, vitamin D, retinyl esters (which may increase in vitamin A toxicity), and a profile of five different carotenoids are being assessed.

Clinical assessments related to nutrition.

Unlike previous NHANES, the physician's examination component of NHANES III did not screen for overt clinical signs of nutritional deficiencies such as keratomalacia, pellagrous dermatitis, or follicular hyperkeratosis, which are uncommon in the United States. Instead, a number of nutrition-related health conditions were assessed in NHANES III (see the section "Health status assessment"), including cardiovascular disease and related risk factors, diabetes, osteoporosis, dental conditions, and gallbladder disease. Dietary and nutrition-related interview information (appendix table X) supplement the physical examination findings and allow for further study of the interrelationships between nutrition and health in the population and subgroups at increased risk.

APPENDIX IV

NHANES-III Summary of Examination & Clinical Biochemistry Assessments and
Dietary/Nutritional Evaluations

(Note: With the exception of the footnote in bold on page IV-8, the material in this Appendix is taken verbatim from the NCHS source document.)

(Source: NCHS, 1994b, pp. 45, 46, 48, 49, 53, 56)

NHANES-III Summary tables

Table 1. Interview topics covered, by type of questionnaire

Household screener	Family questionnaire	Household questionnaires	
		Household adult questionnaire (ages 17 years and over)	*Household youth questionnaire (ages 2 months–16 years)*
Household composition Selection of sample persons Ending interview	Individual characteristics Health insurance and income assistance Family background Occupation of family head Housing characteristics Family characteristics	Blood pressure measurement Orientation Health services Selected conditions Diabetes High blood pressure/cholesterol Cardiovascular disease Musculoskeletal conditions (ages 20 years and over) Gallbladder disease Kidney conditions Respiratory and allergy Diet and body weight Food frequency Vision and hearing Dental care and status Tobacco Physical functioning (ages 60 years and over only during Phase 1) Vision and hearing Occupation/language usage Exercise Social support/residence Vitamin, mineral, and medicine usage Name/Social Security number	Birth (2 months–11 years) Infant feeding practices/diet (2 months– 11 years) Motor and social development Health services and functional impairment Selected conditions Respiratory and allergy Vision and hearing School attendance and language usage Vitamin, mineral, and medicine usage Name/Social Security number Dental care and status

Table 1. Interview topics covered, by type of questionnaire (continued)

Supplemental Questionnaires

MEC Adult Questionnaire (ages 17 years and over)	MEC Youth Questionnaire (ages 8-16 years)	MEC Proxy Questionnaire (ages 2 months - 11years)	Home Examination Questionnaire (ages 2-11 months and 20 years and over)
Tobacco Selected conditions Medicine, vitamin, and mineral usage Cognitive function (ages 60 years and over) Alcohol/drug use Reproductive health Diagnostic interview schedule (ages 17-39 years)	Activity Tobacco Reproductive health (boys ages 12-16 years and girls ages 10-16 years) Selected conditions Medicine, vitamin, and mineral usage (ages 12-16 years) Food frequency (ages 12-16 years) Alcohol/drug use (ages 12-16 years) Diagnostic interview schedule (ages 15-16 years)	Medicine, vitamin, and mineral usage (ages 1-11 years) Selected conditions Infant food frequency (ages 2-11 months)	Infant food frequency (ages 2-11 months) Cognitive function (ages 60 years & over) Selected conditions Medicine, vitamin, and mineral usage (ages 20 years and over) Tobacco Reproductive health (ages 20 years and over)

NOTE: MEC is mobile examination center.

Table 2. Examination components, by age group

2 months–5 years	6-19 years	20-39 years	40-59 years	60-74 years	75 years and over
Physician's exam	Physician's exam	Physician's exam	Physician's exam	Physician's exam	Physician's exam
Dental exam[1]	Dental exam	Dental exam	Dental exam	Dental exam	Dental exam
Body measurements[2]	Body measurements	Body measurements[2]	Body measurements[2]	Body measurements[2]	Body measurements[2]
Venipuncture[1]	Venipuncture	Venipuncture[2]	Venipuncture[2]	Venipuncture[2]	Venipuncture[2]
Dietary interview	Dietary interview	Dietary interview	Dietary interview	Dietary interview	Dietary interview
Health interview	Health interview	Health interview	Health interview	Health interview	Health interview
	Urine collection	Urine collection	Urine collection	Urine collection	Urine collection
	Spirometry[3]	Spirometry[2]	Spirometry[2]	Spirometry[2]	Spirometry[2]
	Bioelectrical impedance[4]	Bioelectrical impedance	Bioelectrical impedance	Bioelectrical impedance	Bioelectrical impedance
	Allergy test	Allergy test[5]	Allergy test[5]	...	...
	Audiometry	...	...	...	...
	Tympanometry	...	...	...	...
	Cognitive test[6]	...	...	Cognitive test[2]	Cognitive test[2]
		Bone density exam	Bone density exam	Bone density exam	Bone density exam
		Ultrasound exam	Ultrasound exam	Ultrasound exam	...
		CNS test[5]	CNS test[5]	...	...
			Fundus photography	Fundus photography	Fundus photography
			Electrocardiography	Electrocardiography	Electrocardiography
				Performance test[2]	Performance test[2]
				Hand/knee x-rays	Hand/knee x-rays

[1] one year of age and over.
[2] Also included in the home examination.
[3] 8 years of age and over.
[4] 12 years of age and over.
[5] Half-sample only.
[6] 6-16 years of age.

NOTE: CNS is central nervous system

IV-4

Table 3. Blood and urine assessments, by age group

	Age Group				
	1-3 years	4-5 years	6-11 years	12-19 years	20 years and over
Whole blood	CBC[1]/RDW Platelets 3-cell differential Differential smear Lead[5] Protoporphyrin[5]	CBC[1]/RDW Platelets 3-cell differential Differential smear Lead[5] Protoporphyrin[5] Red blood cell folate Glycated hemoglobin[5] (Hb A1c)	CBC[1]/RDW Platelets 3-cell differential Differential smear Lead[5] Protoporphyrin[5] Red blood cell folate Glycated hemoglobin[5] (Hb A1c)	CBC[1]/RDW Platelets 3-cell differential Differential smear Lead[5] Protoporphyrin[5] Red blood cell folate Glycated hemoglobin[5] (Hb A1c)	CBC[1]/RDW Platelets 3-cell differential Differential smear Lead[5] Protoporphyrin[5] Red blood cell folate Glycated hemoglobin[5] (Hb A1c)
Serum	Iron[5] Total iron binding capacity[5] Ferritin[5]	Iron[5] Total iron binding capacity[5] Ferritin[5] Folate[5] Apolipoprotein A1,B[4,5] Total cholesterol[5] HDL cholesterol[5] Triglycerides[5] Lp(a)[2,5] Continine C-reactive protein[5] Rheumatoid factor Vitamin A (retinol)[5] Carotenoids[5] Retinyl esters[5] Vitamin E[5] Vitamin B12[2] Methyl malonic acid[2] Homocysteine[2] Helicobacter pylori[4] Tetanus	Iron[5] Total iron binding capacity[5] Ferritin[5] Folate[5] Apolipoprotein A1,B[4,5] Total cholesterol[5] HDL cholesterol[5] Triglycerides[5] Lp(a)[2,5] Continine C-reactive protein[5] Rheumatoid factor Vitamin A (retinol)[5] Carotenoids[5] Retinyl esters[5] Vitamin E[5] Vitamin B12[2] Methyl malonic acid[2] Homocysteine[2] Helicobacter pylori[4] Tetanus Hantavirus (ages 10+)[4] Vitamin C Hepatitis A Hepatitis B/delta Hepatitis C Hepatitis E Rubella[5] Varicella Diphtheria	Iron[5] Total iron binding capacity[5] Ferritin[5] Folate[5] Apolipoprotein A1,B[4,5] Total cholesterol[5] HDL cholesterol[5] Triglycerides[5] Lp(a)[2,5] Continine C-reactive protein[5] Rheumatoid factor Vitamin A (retinol)[5] Carotenoids[5] Retinyl esters[5] Vitamin E[5] Vitamin B12[2] Methyl malonic acid[2] Homocysteine[2] Helicobacter pylori[4] Tetanus Hantavirus[4] Vitamin C Hepatitis A Hepatitis B/delta Hepatitis C Hepatitis E Rubella[5] Varicella Diphtheria Herpes simplex I and II	Iron Total iron binding capacity[5] Ferritin[5] Folate[5] Apolipoprotein A1,B[4,5] Total cholesterol[5] HDL cholesterol[5] Triglycerides[5] Lp(a)[2,5] Continine C-reactive protein[5] Rheumatoid factor Vitamin A (retinol)[5] Carotenoids[5] Retinyl esters[5] Vitamin E[5] Vitamin B12[2] Methyl malonic acid[2] Homocysteine[2] Tetanus Hantavirus[4] Vitamin C Hepatitis A Hepatitis B/delta Hepatitis C Hepatitis E Rubella[5] Varicella Diphtheria Herpes simplex I and II

Table 3. Blood and urine assessments, by age group (continued)

	1-3 years	4-5 years	6-11 years	12-19 years	20 years and over
Age Group				HIV 1 (ages 18+)[3,5]	HIV 1[3,5]
Serum (continued)				Toxoplasmosis[5] Vitamin D (25-hydroxyvitamin D₃) Total/ionized calcium Selenium[5] Thyroxine (T₄) Thyroid-stimulating hormone (TSH) Antithyroglobulin antibodies Antimicrosomal antibodies Biochemistry profile[5] 　Total carbon dioxide 　Blood urea nitrogen 　Total bilirubin 　Alkaline phosphatase 　Total cholesterol 　AST (SGOT) 　ALT (SGPT) 　LDH	Toxoplasmosis[5] Vitamin D (25-hydroxyvitamin D₃) Total/ionized calcium Selenium[5] Thyroxine (T₄) Thyroid-stimulating hormone (TSH) Antithyroglobulin antibodies Antimicrosomal antibodies FSH/LH (females ages 35-60 years) Insulin C-peptide Biochemistry profile[5] 　Total carbon dioxide 　Blood urea nitrogen 　Total bilirubin 　Alkaline phosphatase 　Total cholesterol 　AST (SGOT) 　ALT (SGPT) 　LDH

Table 3. Blood and urine assessments, by age group (continued)

Age group				
1-3 years	4-5 years	6-11 years	12-19 years	20 years and over
Serum (continued)				
			GGT Total protein Albumin Creatinine Glucose Calcium Chloride Uric acid Phosphorus Sodium Potassium	GGT Total protein Albumin Creatinine Glucose Calcium Chloride Uric acid Phosphorus Sodium Potassium
Plasma				
				Glucose (ages 20-39 years, 75 years and over) OGITT (ages 40-74 years) Fibrinogen (ages 40 years and over)[5]
Urine				
		Cadmium Creatinine Albumin (micro) Iodine	Cadmium Creatinine Albumin (micro) Iodine Cocaine[2,3] (ages 18 years and over) Opiates[2,3] (ages 18 years and over) Phencyclidine[2,3] (ages 18 years and over) Amphetamines[2,3] (ages 18 years and over) Marijuana[2,3] (ages 18 years and over)	Cadmium Creatinine Albumin (micro) Iodine Cocaine[2,3] Opiates[2,3] Phencyclidine[2,3] Amphetamines[2,3] Marijuana[2,3] Pregnancy test (females ages 20-59 years)
White cells				
			Storage/banking[5]	Storage/banking[5]

[1] Includes hematocrit, hemoglobin, red and white cell counts, mean corpuscular volume, mean corpuscular hemoglobin, and mean corpuscular hemoglobin concentration.
[2] Phase 2 only.
[3] Anonymous.
[4] Phase 1 only.
[5] Home examination also.

IV-7

Table 4. Special studies

Volatile organic compounds (VOC's)[1]

Benzene	1,1-Dichloroethane	Methylene Chloride
Toluene	1,2-Dichloroethane	Chloroform
Styrene	1,1-Dichloroethene	Carbon Tetrachloride
Ethylbenzene	cis-1,2-Dichlorethene	1,2-Dichloropropane
o-Xylene	trans-1,2-Dichlorethene	Bromoform
m-Xylene	1,1,1-Trichloroethane	Dibromomethane
p-Xylene	1,1,2-Trichloroethane	Bromodichloromethane
Chlorobenzene	Trichloroethene	Dibromochloromethane
1,2-Dichlorobenzene	1,1,2,2-Tetrachloroethane	Acetone
1,3-Dichlorobenzene	Tetrachloroethene	2-Butanone
1,4-Dichlorobenzene	Hexachloroethane	

Pesticides or metabolites[1]

2,4-Dichlorophenol	Pentachlorophenol	2-Isopropoxyphenol
2,5-Dichlorophenol	4-Nitrophenol	Carbofuranphenol
2,4,5-Trichlorophenol	1-Naphthol	3,5,6-Trichloro-2-pyridinol
2,4,6-Trichlorophenol	2-Naphthol	2,4-Dichlorophenoxyacetic-acid

Osteocalcin and bone alkaline phosphatase[2]

High-density lipoprotein phospholipid[3]

Dehydroepiandrosterone[4]

[1]This study was conducted by the Division of Environmental Health Laboratory Sciences, National Center for Environmental Health, Centers for Disease Control and Prevention, on volunteers ages 20-59 years.
[2]This study was conducted on those with a Vitamin D assay, an acceptable bone density scan and a serum creatinine level of ≤2.0 mg/dL. Most were examined during a morning session.
[3]This study was conducted on all persons with coronary heart disease (CHD) and on 600 persons without CHD from 12 age-sex groups.
[4]This study was conducted on 1,400 persons 20-90 years of age from 14 age-sex groups.

NOTE: Data from these studies are not from probability samples and may not be available for public use.

(NOTE: The VOCs were tested in the blood of a random sample of 1,000 subjects. The pesticides were to be tested in the urine of a random sample of 1,000 subjects. Although several NCHS documents indicate that the pesticide testing was conducted, it actually was not; therefore, no data are available for this component).

IV-8

Table 5. Nutrition-Related Interview Information Collected in Interviews, by Age of Sample Person and Type of Information

Information	Age
24-hour dietary recall	2 months and over
Food security[1]	2 months and over
Food program participation[1]	2 months and over
Drinking water source and quantity[1]	2 months and over
Vitamin and mineral supplement usage	2 months and over
Salt use frequency and type	2 months and over
Infant food frequency	2-11 months
Breakfast practices	1 year and over
Dietary changes for health reasons	1 year and over
Infant feeding practices, including breast feeding	2 months -5 years
Food frequency	12 years and over
Alcohol use	12 years and over
Antacids use	17 years and over
Lifetime milk frequency	20 years and over
Self-(or proxy-) reported height and weight	2 months and over
Self-(-or proxy) assessed weight status	2 months and over
Birth weight	2 months - 11 years
Weight loss practices and reasons	1 year and over
Desired weight	12 years and over
Weight history	25 years and over

[1] Also collected at the household (family) level.

APPENDIX V

Comparison of Laboratory Analyses of Blood and Urine Across NHANES-I, -II, -III, and Hispanic HANES

(Note: With the exception of minor changes to the table footnotes, the material in this Appendix is taken verbatim from the NCHS source document.)

(Source: NCHS, 1994b)

Table 1. Comparison of Laboratory Analyses of Blood and Urine Across NHANES-I, -II, -III and Hispanic HANES

Lab Test	SURVEY[1]			
	I	II	HH	III
Whole Blood Assessments:				
Sedimentation rate	x			
Complete blood count	x	x	x	x
Platelets				x
3-cell differential				x
Differential smear	x	x	x	x
Red cell distribution width				x
Lead		x	x	x
Protoporphyrin		x	x	x
Red blood cell folate		x	x	x
Glycated hemoglobin (Hb_{A1c})				x
Carboxyhemoglobin		x	x	
Serum Biochemistry Assessments:				
Folate	x	x	x	x
Iron & total iron-binding capacity	x	x	x	x
Ferritin		x	x	x
Vitamin C		x		x
Vitamin D				x
Vitamin E			x	x
Zinc & copper		x		
Vitamin A (retinol)	x	x[2]	x	x
Carotenoids				x
Retinyl esters				x
Vitamin B12		x		x[3]
Methyl malonic acid				x[3]
Homocysteine				x[3]
Selenium				x
Total cholesterol	x	x	x	x
High density lipoprotein cholesterol		x	x	x
Triglycerides		x	x	x
Apolipoproteins A_1 & B				x[4]
Lp(a)				x[3]
Total & ionized calcium				x
Cotinine				x
Bile salts		x		
Pesticides[7]		x	x	x
Syphilis	x	x	x	
Hepatitis A, B & delta		x	x	x
Hepatitis C			x	x
Hepatitis E			x	x
Tetanus	x		x	x
Diphtheria	x			x
Polio	x			
Herpes simplex I & II		x		x

Lab Test	I	II	HH	III
Serum Biochemistry Assessments:				
Human immunodeficiency virus I				X
Rubella antibody	X			X
Varicella antibody				X
Toxoplasmosis antibody				X
Helicobacter pylori				X[4]
Hantavirus				X[4]
C-reactive protein				X
Rheumatoid factor				X
FSH/LH[5]				X
Thyroxine (T_4)				X
Thyroid-stimulating hormone (TSH)				X
Antithyroglobulin antibodies				X
Antimicrosomal antibodies				X
Insulin				X
C-peptide				X
Biochemistry Profile:				
Total carbon dioxide			X	X
Blood urea nitrogen	X		X	X
Total bilirubin	X	X[6]	X	X
Alkaline phosphatase	X	X[6]	X	X
Total cholesterol	X		X	X
Aspartate aminotransferase (serum glutamic-oxaloacetic transaminase)	X[6]	X[6]	X	X
Alanine aminotransferase (serum glutamate pyruvate transaminase)			X	X
Lactate dehydrogenase			X	X
Gamma glutamyl transpeptidase				X
Total protein	X		X	X
Albumin	X	X	X	X
Creatinine	X	X	X	X
Glucose			X	X
Calcium	X		X	X
Chloride			X	X
Uric acid	X		X	X
Phosphorus	X		X	X
Sodium	X		X	X
Potassium	X		X	X
Plasma Assessments:				
Plasma fibrinogen				X
Glucose (oral glucose tolerance test)		X	X	X

Lab Test	SURVEY[1]			
	I	II	HH	III
Urinary Assessments:				
Urinalysis	x	x	x	
Pesticides[7]		x	x	
Riboflavin	x			
Thiamine	x			
Cadmium				x
Creatinine	x			x
Albumin (micro)				x
Iodine	x			x
Cocaine				x[3]
Opiates				x[3]
Phencyclidine				x[3]
Amphetamines				x[3]
Marijuana				x[3]
Sodium				x
Pregnancy test	x			x
Excess and Reserve Vials				
Serum	x	x	x	x
White blood cells for DNA banking				x

(1) I is NHANES-I, II is NHANES-II, III is NHANES-III and HH is the Hispanic Health and Nutrition Survey

(2) Children only

(3) Phase 2 subjects only

(4) Phase 1 subjects only

(5) Follicle-stimulating hormone/Luteinizing hormone

(6) Bile salts subset

(7) See Table 1 in Appendix VII of this Handbook

APPENDIX VI

Comparison of Laboratory Analyses, Examinations and Questionnaires Across NHANES-99, -00, -01, and -02

(Note: The material in this Appendix is taken verbatim from the NCHS source document. Footnotes were added for clarification as indicated in each table.)

(Source: NHANES Consortium Meeting, 2002)

Table 1. Laboratory Analyses of Blood, Urine and Hair for NHANES-99 to- 02

Lab Test	Age Range	YEAR OF SURVEY			
		1999	2000	2001	2002
Lead [1]	1 year & older	x	x	x	x
Cadmium [1]	1 year & older	x	x	x	x
Erythrocyte protoporphyrin	1 year & older	x	x	x	x
Red blood cell folate	3 years & older	x	x	x	x
Serum folate	3 years & older	x	x	x	x
Glycohemoglobin	12 years & older	x	x	x	x
Mercury (hair)[1]	1- 5 years & females 16-49	x	x	x	
Mercury (blood)[1]	1- 5 years & females 16-49	x	x	x	x
Mercury (urine)[1]	1- 5 years & females 16-49	x	x	x	x
CD4[2]	18 - 49 years	x	x	x	x
White blood cells/DNA	20 years & older	x	x	x	x
Iron	1 year & older	x	x	x	x
TIBC[3]	1 year & older	x	x	x	x
Ferritin	1 year & older	x	x	x	x
Vitamin B12	3 years & older	x	x	x	x
C-Reactive protein	3 years & older	x	x	x	x
Helicobacter pylori	3 years & older	x	x	x	
Cryptosporidium	6 - 49 years	x	x	x	
Vitamin A/E/Carotenoids	3 years & older	x	x	x	x
Vitamin C	6 years & older				
Measles/Varicella/Rubella	6 - 49 years	x	x	x	x
Cotinine	3 years & older	x	x	x	x
Chemistry panel	12 years & older	x	x	x	x
Bone alkaline phosphatase	8 years & older	x	x	x	x
Toxoplasma[4]	6 - 49 years	x	x	x	x
Total cholesterol	3 years & older	x	x	x	x
High density lipoprotein	3 years & older	x	x	x	x
Low density lipoprotein	Subsample 3 years & older	x	x	x	x
Triglycerides	Subsample 3 years & older	x	x	x	x
HIV antibody	18 - 49 years	x	x	x	x
Insulin/c-peptide	Subsample 12 years & older	x	x	x	x
Herpes 1 & 2 antibody	14 - 49 years	x	x	x	x
Syphilis	18 - 49 years			x	x
Human papiloma virus	14 - 59 years				x
Prostate specific antigen	males 40 years & older			x	x
FSH/LH[5]	females 35 - 60 years	x	x	x	x
Latex	12 - 59 years	x	x	x	
Vitamin D	6 years & older		x	x	x
TSH/TH[6]	1/3 subsample 12 years & older	x	x	x	x
EPA persistent pesticides[1]	1/3 subsample 6 years & older	x	x	x	x
surplus sera	6 years & older	x	x	x	x
Homocysteine	3 years & older	x	x	x	x
Methyl malonic acid	3 years & older	x	x	x	x

		YEAR OF SURVEY			
Lab Test	**Age Range**	**1999**	**2000**	**2001**	**2002**
Glucose (plasma)	Subsample 12 years & older	x	x	x	x
Fibrinogen	40 years & older	x	x	x	x
Hepatitis B antibodies	2 - 5 years	x	x	x	x
Hepatitis A, B, C, D HbSAg	6 years & older	x	x	x	x
Complete blood count	1year & older	x	x	x	x
Selenium	3 - 11 years	x	x	x	
Chlamydia (urine)	14 - 39 years	x	x	x	x
Gonorrhea (urine)	14 - 39 years	x	x	x	x
Albumin (urine)	6 years & older	x	x	x	x
Creatinine (urine)	6 years & older	x	x	x	x
NTX[7]	8 years & older	x	x	x	x
Iodine (urine)	1/3 sample 6 years & older	x	x	x	x
BV/Trich[8]	Females 14 - 49 years			x	x
MRSA[9]	1 year & older			x	x
VOC[10] exposure monitor[1]	Subsample 20 - 59 years	x	x	x	
Pthalates[1]	1/3 subsample 6 years & older	x	x	x	x
OP metabolites[1, 11]	1/3 subsample 6 years & older	x	x	x	x
Metals[1]	1/3 subsample 6 years & older	x	x	x	x
Nonpersistent pesticides-LC[1]	1/3 subsample 12 - 19 years	x	x	x	x
Nonpersistent pesticides-GC[1]	1/3 subsample 12 years & older	x	x	x	x
Phytoestrogens[1]	1/3 subsample 6 years & older	x	x	x	x
PAHs[1, 12]	1/3 subsample 6 years & older	x	x	x	x
Dioxins[1]	1/3 subsample 12 years & older	x	x	x	x
Lead dust[1]	Households with 1 - 5 year olds	x	x	x	x
VOC (blood)[1, 10]	Subsample 20 - 59 years	x	x	x	x

(Sources: Table was presented at the 2002 NCHS Consortium meeting of the NHANES sponsoring agencies; several footnotes were generated based on information in NCHS, 2001.)

(1) See Table 1 from Appendix VII of this Handbook

(2) In addition to HIV testing in NHANES-99+, whole blood samples will be collected and stored for future CD4 testing once the HIV status of the subject is known. This will allow for the determination of the distribution of CD4 cells in a random sample of HIV positive individuals.

(3) TIBC is Total Iron Binding Capacity.

(4) Surplus sera used for years 1999 and 2000.

(5) Follicle-stimulating hormone/Luteinizing hormone

(6) Thyroid-stimulating hormone/Thyroxine

(7) NTX is a marker in the urine indicative of bone mineral resorption. It is used in conjunction with bone alkaline phosphatase (a marker in the serum for bone formation) to evaluate a subject's bone mineral status.

(8) BV/Trich are bacterial vaginosis and Trichomoniasis. Both are tested by using vaginal swabs.

(9) MRSA is methicillin-resistant *Staph aureus*. Nasal swabs will be tested for this bacterium.

(10) VOCs are volatile organic compounds.

(11) OP is organophosphate pesticide.

(12) PAH is polyaromatic hydrocarbon.

Table 2. Questionnaire Matrix for NHANES-99 to -02

Component	Age Range[1]	YEAR OF SURVEY			
		1999	2000	2001	2002
Subject Questionnaire:					
Acculturation	12 years & older	x	x	x	x
Audiometry	20 years & older	x	x	x	x
Balance	40 years & older	x	x	x	x
Hospital utilization & access to health care	0 years & older	x	x	x	x
Blood pressure	16 years & older	x	x	x	x
Cardiovascular diseases	40 years & older	x	x	x	x
Demographics	0 years & older	x	x	x	x
Dermatology	6 years & older	x	x	x	x
Diabetes	1 year & older	x	x	x	x
Diet behavior & nutrition	0 years & older	x	x	x	x
Dietary supplements & medications	0 years & older	x	x	x	x
Digit Symbol Substitution Test[2]	60 years & older	x	x	x	x
Early childhood	0 - 15 years	x	x	x	x
Immunizations	0 years & older	x	x	x	x
Introduction & verification	0 years & older	x	x	x	x
Kidney conditions	20 years & older	x	x	x	x
Medical conditions	1 year & older	x	x	x	x
Miscellaneous pain	20 years & older	x	x	x	x
Occupation	12 years & older	x	x	x	x
Oral health	2 years & older	x	x	x	x
Osteoporosis	20 years & older	x	x	x	x
Physical activity & physical fitness	2 years & older	x	x	x	x
Physical functioning	1 year & older	x	x	x	x
Respiratory health & disease	1 year & older	x	x	x	x
Smoking & tobacco use	20 years & older	x	x	x	x
Social support	60 years & older	x	x	x	x
Tuberculosis	1 year & older	x	x		
Vision	20 years & older	x	x	x	x
Weight history	16 years & older	x	x	x	x
Family Questionnaire:					
Demographic background/Occupation	0 years & older	x	x	x	x
Food security	0 years & older	x	x	x	x
Health insurance	0 years & older	x	x	x	x
Housing characteristics	0 years & older	x	x	x	x
Income	0 years & older	x	x	x	x
Pesticide use	0 years & older	x	x	x	x
Smoking	0 years & older	x	x	x	x
Tracking & tracing	0 years & older	x	x	x	x

(Sources: Table was presented at the 2002 NCHS Consortium meeting of the NHANES sponsoring agencies; footnote #2 was generated based on information in NCHS, 2001b.)

(1) Age range of subjects varies for specific components within each of the specified sections.

(2) Digit Symbol Substitution Test requires the subject to correctly code a series of symbols in 120 seconds. This exercise is used as a sensitive measure of dementia, and requires response speed, sustained attention, visual spatial skills, associative learning, and memory.

Table 3. Examination Matrix for NHANES-99 to -02

Component	Age Range	1999	2000	2001	2002
		YEAR OF SURVEY			
Audiometry	half sample 20-69 years	x	x	x	x
Balance	see footnote (1)			x	x
BIA[2]	8 - 49 years	x	x	x	x
Body measures (anthropometry)[3]	all ages	x	x	x	x
Cardiovascular fitness	12 - 49 years	x	x	x	x
DXA[4]	see footnote (4)		x	x	x
Dietary[5]	all ages	x	x	x	x[5]
Lower Extremity Disease	40 years & older	x	x	x	x
Peripheral vascular disease	40 years & older	x	x	x	x
Peripheral neuropathy	40 years & older	x	x	x	x
Muscle strength	50 years & older	x	x	x	x
Vision	12 years & older	x	x	x	x
Oral health	2 years & older	x	x	x	x
Physician's exam	all ages	x	x	x	x
Blood pressure	8 years & older	x	x	x	x
Sexually transmitted diseases	14 - 49 years	x	x	x	x
BV/Trich[6]	14 - 49 years			x	x
Syphilis	18 - 49 years			x	x
PSA (prostate-specific antigen)	males 40 years & over			x	x
HPV(human papiloma virus)	females 14 -59 years				x
TB (tuberculin) testing	1 year & older	x	x		
VOC badge	subsample 20 - 59 years	x	x	x	
Hair mercury	1 - 5 years; females 16-49	x	x	x	
MRSA[7]	1 year & older			x	x
Hepatitis C follow-up	all subjects w/Hepatitis C			x	x
Dermatology exam[8]	20 - 59 years				x[8]
MEC interview	12 years & older	x	x	x	x
CAPI[9]	12 years & older	x	x	x	x
Physical activity	12 - 15 years	x	x	x	x
Current health status	12 years & older	x	x	x	x
Tobacco use	20 years & older	x	x	x	x
Alcohol use	20 years & older	x	x	x	x
Reproductive health	12 years & older	x	x	x	x
Kidney-urogenital health	20 years & older	x	x	x	x
ACASI[10]	12 years & older	x	x	x	x
Sexual behavior	14 - 59 years	x	x	x	x
Drug use	14 - 59 years	x	x	x	x
Tobacco use	12 - 19 years	x	x	x	x
Alcohol use	12 - 19 years	x	x	x	x
Youth conduct disorder	12 - 19 years	x	x	x	x
Urologic health & PSA	males 20 years & older			x	x
Mental health questions	8 - 39 years	x	x	x	x

(Sources: Table was presented at the 2002 NCHS Consortium meeting of the NHANES sponsoring agencies; several footnotes were generated based on information in NCHS, 2001and 2001a.)

(1) MEC locations 101-124 tested a half sample of subjects 40-69 years. Locations 125 and beyond will test individuals 40 years and older.

(2) BIA is bioelectrical impedance analysis and is a clinical method for measuring impedance of body tissues. The resulting information provides data on body composition, including lean and fat tissue.

(3) Body measures include weight, stature, recumbent length, lengths and circumferences of body parts, and skinfold measures.

(4) DXA is dual-energy X-ray absorptiometry and is a clinical method for measuring body composition (bone, lean and fat tissue). DXA provides information on bone density and soft tissue composition. MEC locations 101-112 tested males 8 years and older and females 18 years and older. Locations 113 and beyond will test subjects 8 years and older.

(5) A new dietary interview was started in 2002 and included a 2nd day recall by phone interview.

(6) BV/Trich are bacterial vaginosis and Trichomoniasis. Both are tested by using vaginal swabs.

(7) MRSA is methicillin-resistant *Staph aureus*. Nasal swabs will be tested for this bacterium.

(8) The dermatology exam will be pilot tested in 2002, and will go into field in 2003.

(9) CAPI is Computer-Assisted Personal Interviewing. Randomly selected people are invited to participate in NHANES-99+ by first being interviewed in their homes. Household interview data are collected via CAPI and include demographic, socioeconomic, dietary, and health-related questions. After completion of the interview, respondents are asked to participate in a physical examination at the MEC.

(10) ACASI is Audio-Computer-Assisted-Self-Interviewing (CASI)system, and is generally used for sensitive topic areas. Subjects listen to a recorded voice though a headset, as well as reading the questions on the screen, and then indicate their response by touching the computer screen. ACASI is conducted at the MEC.

APPENDIX VII

Comparison of Environmental Data Collected Across all NHANES

(Sources: NCHS, 1973, 1977, 1981, 1985, 1994b; NCHS website: <http://www.cdc.gov/nchs/about/major/nhanes/questexam.htm> for *Survey Questionnaires, Examination Components and Laboratory Components* for NHANES 99+)

Table 1. Comparison of Key Environmental Data Collected Across the NHANES Surveys

	NHANES I 1971-1975	NHANES II 1976-1980	HHANES 1982-1984	NHANES III 1988-1994	NHANES 99+ (1999-indefinitely)
BLOOD AND SERUM					
Cadmium	No	No	No	No	1+ yrs
Carboxyhemoglobin	No	SPs 3-74 yrs (½ sample)	SPs 3-74 yrs (½ sample in the first yr)	No	No
Cotinine[1]	No	No	No	SPs 4-74+ yrs	SPs 3+ yrs
Dioxins, Furans, Coplanar PCBs[2]	No	No	No	No	SPs 12+ yrs (1/3 sample)
Lead	No	all children 6 mo - 6 yrs; & SPs 7-74 yrs (½ sample)	SPs 6 mo-74 yrs	SPs 1-74+ yrs	SPs 1+ yrs
Mercury[3]	No	No	No	No	All SPs 1-5 yrs & women 16-49 yrs
PCBs[4]	No	No	all SPs 12-19 yrs & SPs 20-74 yrs (½ sample)	No	SPs 12+ yrs (1/3 sample)
Pesticide residues & metabolites[5]	No	SPs 12-19 yrs (½ sample) & all SPs 20-74 yrs	all SPs 12-19 yrs & SPs 20-74 yrs (½ sample)	No	SPs 12+ yrs (1/3 sample)
Phytoestrogens[6]	No	No	No	No	SPs 12+ yrs (1/3 sample)
Volatile Organic Compounds (VOCs)[7]	No	No	No	non-random subsample of 1000 SPs 20-59 yrs	random subsample each year of 1000 SPs 20-59 yrs
URINE					
Cadmium	No	No	No	SPs 6-74+ yrs	SPs 6+ yrs (1/3 sample)

Heavy Metals (other than Cadmium)[8]	No	No	No	No	SPs 6+ yrs (1/3 sample)
Organophosphates Pesticide Screen[9]	No	No	No	No	SPs 6-11 yrs (½ sample) & 12+ yrs (1/4 sample)
Pesticide residues & metabolites[10]	No	SPs 12-74 yrs (½ sample)	SPs 12-74 yrs (½ sample)	1000 SPs ages 20-59 yrs were to be tested for several pesticides but were not	SPs 6-11 yrs (½ sample) & 12+ yrs (1/4 sample)
Phthalates[11]	No	No	No	No	SPs 6+ yrs (1/3 sample)
Phytoestrogens[6]	No	No	No	No	SPs 6+ yrs (1/3 sample)
Polyaromatic Hydrocarbons (PAHs)[12]	No	No	No	No	SPs 6+ yrs (1/3 sample)
OTHER					
Lead dust in homes[13]	No	No	No	No	Households with SPs 1-5 yrs
Household water samples[14]	trace minerals drinking water 3059 SPs 25-74 yrs	No	No	No	VOCs from home tap water of a random subsample of 1000 SPs 20-59 yrs
Hair[15]	No	No	All SPs ages 12-74 for selected trace metals for a CDC pilot study	No	All SPs 1-5 yrs & women 16-49 yrs, for total mercury
Personal Smoking & Environmental Tobacco Smoke Questions[16]	SPs 25-74 yrs	SPs 12-74 yrs	SPs 12-74 yrs	SPs 8+ yrs.	All SPs
Pesticide Exposure (Self-reported)[17]	No	SPs 12-74 yrs	SPs 12-74 yrs	No	Use of pesticides in home & yard

[1]Cotinine is a metabolic byproduct of nicotine metabolism. Cotinine levels and other data (i.e., self-reported

VII-3

smoking and exposure to others who smoke) gathered in NHANES-III and NHANES99+ can be used to help assess: 1) prevalence and extent of tobacco use in subjects; 2) extent of exposure to environmental tobacco smoke (ETS), and determine trends in exposure to ETS; and 3) relationships between tobacco use (and/or ETS) and chronic health conditions (e.g., respiratory and cardiovascular diseases).

[2] NHANES99+ tested for the following dioxins, furans and coplanar PCBs in serum: 2,3,7,8-Tetrachloro-dibenzo-p-dioxin (tcdd); 1,2,3,7,8-Pentachloro-dibenzo-p-dioxin (pncdd); 1,2,3,4,7,8-Hexachloro-dibenzo-p-dioxin (hxcdd); 1,2,3,6,7,8-Hexachloro-dibenzo-p-dioxin (hxcdd); 1,2,3,7,8,9-Hexachloro-dibenzo-p-dioxin (hxcdd); 1,2,3,4,6,7,8-Heptachloro-dibenzo-p-dioxin (hpcdd); 1,2,3,4,6,7,9-Heptachloro-dibenzo-p-dioxin (hpcdd); 1,2,3,4,6,7,8,9-Octachloro-dibenzo-p-dioxin (ocdd); 2,3,7,8-Tetrachloro-dibenzofuran (tcdf); 1,2,3,7,8-Pentachloro-dibenzofuran (pncdf).

[3] In NHANES99+, mercury was tested in the blood, hair and urine of this subsample of women and children.

[4] HHANES did not identify specific PCBs that were tested. NHANES99+ tested for the following noncoplanar PBCs in serum: PCB-19, 28, 44, 49, 52, 56, 60, 66, 74, 87, 99, 101, 105, 110, 116, 118, 128, 138, 146, 149.

[5] Pesticide residues and metabolites in blood or serum for NHANES-II, HHANES, and NHANES99+: aldrin, *beta*-BHC, *gamma*-BHC, op'-DDD, pp'-DDD, op'-DDE, pp'-DDE, op'-DDT, dieldrin, endrin, heptachlor epoxide, hexachlorobenzene, mirex, oxychlordane, *trans*-Nonachlor. NHANES-II and HHANES (but not NHANES99+) also tested for *alpha*-BHC, delta-BHC,pp'-DDT, heptachlor.
Additional pesticide residues and metabolites tested in blood or serum only in NHANES99+: *alpha*-Chlordane, cis-Nonachlor, *gamma*-Chlordane, Lindane, Nitrobenzene.

[6] Phytoestrogens measured in both serum and urine in NHANES99+ were: Coumestrol, Daidzein, Enterodiol, Enterolactone, Equol, Genistein, Matairesinol, o-Desmethylangolensin (O-DMA).

[7] In NHANES-III, only blood samples were analyzed for selected VOCs. In NHANES99+, personal exposures to VOCs were characterized by testing for chemicals in personal air samples, blood, and drinking water of selected subjects. Air samples were obtained by small lightweight passive sampling badges worn by subjects for 48-hours. Badges were returned to the MEC 48-72 hours later along with a sample of tap water from their homes. Blood samples were taken when the badges were returned. Both NHANES-III and NHANES99+ measured blood levels of the following VOCs: 1,1,1-Trichloroethane; 1,1,2,2-Tetrachloroethane; 1,1,2-Trichloroethane; 1,2-Dichloroethane; 1,2-Dichloropropane; 1,3-Dichlorobenzene; 1,4-Dichlorobenzene; 2-Butanone; Acetone; Benzene; Bromodichloromethane; Bromoform; Carbon Tetrachloride; Chlorobenzene; Chloroform; Dibromochloromethane; Dibromomethane; Ethylbenzene; Hexachloroethane; Xylenes; Methylene chloride; Styrene; Tetrachloroethene; Toluene; Trichloroethene. NHANES99+ also tested blood for the following VOCs that were not tested in NHANES-III: 1,1-Dichloroethane; 1,1-Dichloroethene; 1,2-Dichlorobenzene; cis-1,2-Dichloroethene; Methyl tertiary-butyl ether; trans-1,2-Dichloroethene.

NHANES99+ VOCs measured in both air and blood were: benzene, carbon tetrachloride, chloroform, 1,4-dichlorobenzene, ethyl benzene, methylene chloride, methyl tertiary-butyl ether, styrene, toluene, xylenes, tetrachloroethylene, trichloroethylene. VOCs measured in air but not blood were: 1,3-butadiene.

NHANES99+ VOCs measured in both blood and home water were: Chloroform, Bromodichloromethane, Bromoform, Methyl tertiary-butyl ether, Chlorodibromomethane.

[8] Heavy metals, other than Cd, tested in urine in NHANES99+ were: Antimony, Barium, Beryllium, Cesium, Chromium, Cobalt, Iodine, Lead, Manganese, Mercury (total), Molybdenum, Platinum, Thallium, Thorium, Tin, Tungsten, Uranium.

[9] Organophosphate pesticides in this screen were: Dimethylphosphate, Diethylphosphate, Dimethylthiophosphate,

Diethylthiophosphate, Dimethyldithiophosphate, Diethyldithiophosphate

[10] Pesticide residues and metabolites measured in urine of subjects from NHANES-II, HHANES and NHANES99+ were: 1-Naphthol; 2,4,5-T; 2,4,5-Tricholorphenol; 2,4-D; 2-Isopropoxyphenol; 3,5,6-Trichloropyridinol; Carbofuranphenol; Dicamba; *para*-nitrophenol, Pentachlorophenol.

Additional pesticide residues and metabolites measured in urine from NHANES-II subjects only were: *alpha*-Monocarboxylic acid; Dicarboxylic acid; DMTP, DETP, DMDTP, DEDTP, DMP, and DEP.

Additional pesticide residues and metabolites measured in urine from HHANES subjects only were: Malathion Dicarboxylic Acid and Malathion Monocarboxylic Acid.

Additional pesticide residues and metabolites measured in urine from NHANES99+ subjects only were: 2,4,6-Trichlorophenol; 2,4-Dichlorophenol; 2,5-Dichlorophenol; 2-Naphthol; 3,4-Dichloroaniline; 3-Phenoxy Benzoic Acid; Alachlor Mercapturate; Atrazine Mercapturate; DEET, Glyphosate, Malathion di-acid; Metolachlor Mercapturate; Oxypyrimidine; o-Phenyl phenol.

[11] Phthalates tested in urine were: Bisphenol A; Mono-(2-ethyl)-hexyl phthalate; Mono-benzyl phthalate; Mono-cyclohexyl phthalate; Mono-ethyl phthalate; Mono-isodecyl phthalate; Mono-isononyl phthalate; Mono-n-butyl phthalate; Mono-n-octyl phthalate; Nonyl-phenol; Octyl-phenol.

[12] Polyaromatic hydrocarbons tested in urine were: 1-Hydroxy-aniline; 1-Hydroxy-benzo[b]fluoranthene; 1-Hydroxy-chrysene; 1-Hydroxy-naphthalene; 1-Hydroxy-pyrene; 2-Hydroxy-aniline; 2-Hydroxy-naphthalene; 2-Hydroxy-phenanthrene; 3-Hydroxy-benz[a]anthracene; 3-Hydroxy-benzo[3] pyrene; 3-Hydroxy-benzo[a] pyrene; 3-Hydroxy-benzo[b]fluoranthene; 3-Hydroxy, dibenz [a,h]anthracene; 3-Hydroxy-fluorene; 3-Hydroxy-phenanthrene; Hydroxy-acenaphthalene; Hydroxy-benzo[a]fluoranthene; Hydroxy-benzo[c]phenanthrene; Hydroxy-benzo[g,h]perylene; Hydroxy-benzo[j]fluoranthene; Hydroxy-benzo[k]fluoranthene; Hydroxy-fluoranthene; Hydroxy-indeno[1,2,3-cd]pyrene; Hydroxy-perylene.

[13] In NHANES99+ , window sill and floor dust samples are collected in the home at the time of the household interview. This information can be used to examine the relationship between dust and blood levels, along with other risk factors and housing characteristics.

[14] As part of the NHANES-I Augmentation Survey of Adults 25-74 years of age, water samples were collected from subjects' taps or wells and from public water distribution supplies and tested for hardness, alkalinity, total amount of solute present, and levels of trace minerals. Subjects also were asked numerous questions about personal water consumption, sources of drinking water, and water supplied to the household. This study was conducted to examine possible relationships between hardness and trace minerals in the water and cardiovascular disease.

As part of the special VOC study in NHANES99+ (see footnote #7) VOCs measured in home water were: Chloroform, Bromodichloromethane, Bromoform, Methyl tertiary-butyl ether, Chlorodibromomethane.

[15] The objective of the NHANES99+ hair mercury component was to document total mercury levels in hair, because relationships have been established between the concentrations of mercury in human scalp hair and dietary methylmercury exposure. Hair samples were collected during the first three years of NHANES99+ from males and females aged 1-5 years and females aged 16-49 years.

[16] Personal smoking: NHANES-I, -II asked the same several questions about smoking habits (cigarettes, cigars, pipe, chewing tobacco) of the subjects. NHANES-III subjects ages 8+ yrs , were asked similar questions. All NHANES99+ subjects were asked about personal smoking and those 20+ years old were asked additional, more detailed questions.

Environmental tobacco smoke (ETS): NHANES-III and NHANES99+ inventoried the number of people who smoke in each household and how much each one smokes per day. Additionally in NHANES-III, youths up to 16 yrs old were asked questions about the number of people who smoke cigarettes in the home and how much each one smokes, and subjects 17+ years were also asked about ETS in the workplace. All NHANES99+ subjects were also asked about exposure to ETS at home and at work and in-utero ETS exposure among children.

[17] NHANES-II asks questions about use of pesticides, such as weedkillers, insecticides, fungicides and other chemicals, at the home, in the yard or at work. HHANES asks many questions about subject's work in the farming industry and use of pesticides as part of subject's employment. NHANES99+ asks questions about the use of pesticides in the home and yard.

APPENDIX VIII

ANNOTATED BIBLIOGRAPHY OF STUDIES USING NHANES DATA

(Sources: NCHS, 1996d, 1999b)

Albanes, D; Jones, DY; Micozzi, MS; Mattson ME (1987). Associations between smoking and body weight in the US population: analysis of NHANES II. *Am. J. Pub. Hlth.* 77(4, Apr), 439-444. [adult; aged; body height; body weight; caloric intake; NHANES-II; smoking].

Albanes, D; Jones, DY; Schatzkin, A; Micozzi, MS; Taylor, PR (1988). Adult stature and risk of cancer. *Cancer Res.* 48(6, Mar 15), 1658-1662. [adult; aged; body height; caloric intake; middle age; neoplasms, epidemiology; NHANES-I; nutrition; risk-factors; smoking].

Albanes, D; Blair, A; Taylor, PR (1989). Physical activity and risk of cancer in the NHANES I population. *Am. J. Pub. Hlth.* 79(6, Jun), 744-750. [adult; aged; body constitution; body weight; cohort studies; exercise; health surveys; life style; middle age; neoplasms, epidemiology; NHANES-I; nutrition surveys; recreation; risk-factors].

Anda, RF; Williamson, DF; Escobedo, LG; Remington, PL (1990). Smoking and the risk of peptic ulcer disease among women in the United States. *Arch. Intern. Med.* 150(7, Jul), 1437-1441. [adult; aged; cohort studies; follow-up studies; incidence; middle age; NHANES-I; peptic ulcer, epidemiology; peptic ulcer, etiology; prevalence; risk-factors; sex factors; smoking, adverse effects; United States, epidemiology].

Anderson, LA Jr (1995). A review of blood lead results from the Third National Health and Nutrition Examination Survey (NHANES III). *Am. Ind. Hyg. Assoc. J.* 56(1, Jan), 7-8. [environmental exposure; health surveys; lead poisoning, prevention and control; lead, blood; NHANES III; United States].

Anon. (1989): Iron nutrition and risk of cancer. *Nutr. Rev.* 47(6, June), 176-178.(Includes 11 references.) [iron; nutritional state; nutrient intake; iron binding capacity; carcinoma; risks; epidemiology; nutrition surveys; NHANES-I].

Arnetz, BB; Nicolich, MJ (1990). Modeling of environmental lead contributors to blood lead in human. Int. Arch. *Occup. Env. Hlth.* 62(5), 397-402. [environmental exposure; lead poisoning, epidemiology; NHANES II].

Arrighi, HM; Boyd, BK; Casty, FE (1995). Childhood asthma and adult height: Data from NHANES II. *Pediatric Asthma, Allergy and Immunology* 9(3), 157-163.
[adult; aged; asthma; body height; caucasian; data analysis; education; female; high school; human; major clinical study; male; negro; NHANES II; social status].

Ashley, DL; Bonin, MA; Cardinali, FL; McCraw, JM; Wooten, JV (1994). Blood concentrations of volatile organic compounds in a non-occupational exposed US population and in groups with suspected exposure. *Clin. Chem.* 40(7 Pt 2, Jul), 1401-1404. [environmental exposure; environmental pollutants, blood; NHANES III].

Ballard-Barbash, R; Schatzkin, A; Taylor, PR; Kahle, LL (1990). Association of change in body mass with breast cancer. *Cancer Res.* 50(7, Apr 1), 2152-2155. [alcohol drinking; body weight;

breast neoplasms, etiology; NHANES I; NHEFS].

Ballew, C; Khan, LK; Kaufmann, R; Mokdad, A; Miller, DT; Gunter, EW (1999). Blood lead concentration and children's anthropometric dimensions in the Third National Health and Nutrition Examination Survey (NHANES 111), 1988-1994. *J. Pediatr.* 134 (5, May), 623-630. [blood lead levels; BMI; children; height; Mexican Americans; NHANES-II; NHANES-III; non-Hispanic Blacks; non-Hispanic Whites].
OBJECTIVE: To assess the association between lead exposure and children's physical growth. DESIGN: Cross-sectional analysis of data from the Third National Health and Nutrition Examination Survey, 1988-1994. PARTICIPANTS: A total of 4391 non-Hispanic white, non-Hispanic black, and Mexican-American children age 1 to 7 years. Measurements and Results: We investigated the association between blood lead concentration and stature, head circumference, weight, and body mass index with multiple regression analysis adjusting for sex, ethnic group, iron status, dietary intake, medical history, sociodemographic factors, and household characteristics. Blood lead concentration was significantly negatively associated with stature and head circumference. Regression models predicted reductions of 1.57 cm in stature and 0.52 cm in head circumference for each 0.48 micromol/L (10 micrograms/dL) increase in blood lead concentration. We did not find significant associations between blood lead concentration and weight or body mass index. CONCLUSIONS: The significant negative associations between blood lead concentration and stature and head circumference among children age 1 through 7 years, similar in magnitude to those reported for the Second National Health and Nutrition Examination Survey, 1976-1980, suggest that although mean blood lead concentrations of children have been declining in the United States for 2 decades, lead exposure may continue to affect the growth of some children.

Bang, KM; Gergen, PJ; Carroll, M (1990). Prevalence of chronic bronchitis among US Hispanics from the Hispanic Health and Nutrition Examination Survey, 1982-84. *Am. J. Pub. Hlth.* 80(12, Dec), 1495-1497. [adolescence; bronchitis, epidemiology; HHANES; Hispanic Americans; DHES]

Bang, KM (1993). Prevalence of chronic obstructive pulmonary disease in blacks. *J. Natl. Med. Assoc.* 85(1, Jan), 51-55. [adult; lung diseases, obstructive, epidemiology; negroid race; NHANES I]

Bang, KM; Gergen, PJ; Kramer, R; Cohen, B (1993). The effect of pulmonary impairment on all-cause mortality in a national cohort. *Chest* 103(2, Feb), 536-540. [adult; aged; forced expiratory volume; mortality; NHANES-I; NHEFS; vital capacity; DHES].

Basu, S; Landis JR (1995). Model-based estimation of population attributable risk under cross-sectional sampling. *Am. J. Epid.* 142(12, Dec 15), 1338-1343. [adolescence; adult; cohort studies; models, statistical; NHANES-II]

Berney, B (1993). Round and round it goes: the epidemiology of childhood lead poisoning, 1950-1990. *Milbank. Q.* 71(1), 3-39. [attitude to health; child; child welfare, legislation and jurisprudence; child welfare, trends; health policy, trends; lead poisoning, epidemiology; NHANES-II; public health, trends].

Block ,G (1992). Dietary assessment issues related to cancer for NHANES III. *Vital Health Stat.* 4(27, Mar), 24-31. [case-control studies; cohort studies; cross-sectional studies; data collection, methods; diet records; diet surveys; diet, adverse effects; neoplasms, etiology; NHANES-III; questionnaires]

Briefel, RR (1994). Assessment of the US diet in national nutrition surveys: national collaborative efforts and NHANES. *Am. J. Clin. Nutr.* 59(1 Suppl, Jan), 164S-167S. [adolescence; adult; aged; child; child, preschool; diet; ethnic groups; infant; middle age; NHANES-III; nutrition assessment; nutrition surveys; nutritional status; research design; United States; DHES]

Brody, DJ; Pirkle, JL; Kramer ,RA; Flegal, KM; Matte, TD; Gunter, EW; Paschal, DC (1994). Blood lead levels in the US population. Phase 1 of the third National Health and Nutrition Examination Survey (NHANES III, 1988 to 1991) [see comments]. *JAMA* 272(4, Jul 27), 277-283. [adolescence; adult; age factors; aged; child; child, preschool; cross-sectional studies; health surveys; infant; lead, blood; NHANES III; DHES]

Brody, DJ; Pirkle, JL; Kramer, RA; Flegal, KM; Matte, TD; Gunter, EW; Centers for Disease Control and Prevention (1995): Erratum: Blood lead levels in the US population: Phase 1 of the Third National Health and Nutrition Examination Survey (NHANES III, 1988 to 1991, *JAMA* (1994) 272, 277-283). *JAMA* 274(2), 130. [erratum; error; NHANES III; DHES]

Buckley, TJ; Liddle, J; Ashley, DL; Paschal, DC; Burse, VW; Needham, LL; Akland, G (1997). Environmental and biomarker measurements in nine homes in the Lower Rio Grande Valley: Multimedia results for pesticides, metals, PAHs, and VOCs. *Envir. International* 23, 705-732. [environmental biomarker; NHANES III]
Residential environmental and biomarker measurements were made of multiple pollutants during two seasons (spring and summer, 1993) in order to assess human exposure for a purposeful sample of 18 nonsmoking adults residing within nine homes (a primary and secondary subject in each home) in the Lower Rio Grande Valley (LRGV) near Brownsville, TX. Pesticides, metals, PAHs, VOCs, and PCBs were measured in drinking water, food, air, soil, end house dust over a one- to two-day period in each season. Biomarker measurements were made in blood, breath, and urine. A total of 375 measurements across five pollutant classes (227 pesticides, 44 trace elements, 78 VOCs, 18 PAHs, and 8 PCBs) was possible for each home in one or more media. A large percentage of the measurements was below the method limit of detection ranging from 0-37% for pesticides, 22-61% for metals, 6% and 90% for VOCs in water and air, respectively, and 0-74% for PAHs. The total number of analytes measurable in blood, urine, or breath was considerably less, i.e., 58 (21 pesticides, 1 PCB, 4 metals, 31 VOCs, and 1 PAH) with the percentage above the method limit of detection for pesticides and metals ranging from 40 to 100%, while for VOCs, PAHs, and PCBs, this percentage ranged from 2 to 33%. A significant seasonal difference ($p <$ or $= 0.10$) was found in the biomarker levels of two of seven

nonpersistent pesticides (3,5,6- trichloro-2-pyridinol end 2,5-dichlorophenol) and 3 of 3 metals (arsenic, cadmium, and mercury) and the pyrene metabolite, 1-hydroxypyrene, measured in urine. In all cases, levels were higher in the summer relative to the spring. For the persistent pesticides and PCBs in blood serum, a seasonal effect could be evaluated for 5 of 10 analyzes; a significant difference ($p \leq 0.10$) was observed only for hexachlorobenzene, which like the urine biomarkers, was higher in the summer. In contrast to the urine metals, blood-Pb concentrations did not change significantly ($p <$ or $= 0.05$) from spring to summer. Biological results from the current study are compared to the reference range furnished by the Third National Health and Nutrition Examination Survey (NHANES III). Comparisons are only suggestive due to limitations in comparability between the two studies. Based on the percentage of measurements above the detection limit, a significant elevation ($p \leq 0.10$) in 2 of 12 nonpersistent pesticides (4-nitrophenol and 2,4-D) was observed for the LRGV study subjects. The VOC carbon tetrachloride was found in the blood (monitored only in spring) with greater prevalence ($p \leq 0.10$) than would be expected from NHANES III results. Blood serum levels of two persistent pesticides (4,4'-DDE, and trans-nonachlor) and PCB exceeded median and/or 95th percentile reference levels as did arsenic in urine. Where seasonal differences were identified or for compounds exceeding reference levels, environmental monitoring results were investigated to identify potential contributing pathways and sources of exposure. However, because environmental sampling did not always coincide with the biological sampling and because of the high frequency of analytes measured below the limit of detection, sources and pathways of exposure in many cases could not be explained. Chlorpyrifos was an exception where urine metabolite (3,5,6-TCP) levels were found to be significantly correlated with air ($R2=0.55$; $p \leq 0.01$) and dust ($R2=0.46$; $p \leq 0.01$) concentrations. Based on the results of biomarkers and residential environmental measurements over two seasons, this seeping study shows a seasonal effect for some analytes and suggests where exposures may be high for others. This information may be useful in considering future studies in the region.

Burt, VL; Harris, T (1994). The third National Health and Nutrition Examination Survey: contributing data on aging and health. *Gerontologist* 34(4, Aug), 486-490. [activities of daily living; aged; aged, 80 and over; cardiovascular diseases, epidemiology; health status; health surveys; longitudinal studies; lung diseases, obstructive, epidemiology; musculoskeletal diseases, epidemiology; NHANES-III; nutrition surveys; nutritional status; DHES]

Caraballo, RS; Giovino, GA; Pechacek, TF; Mowery, PD; Richter, PA; Strauss, WJ; Sharp, DJ; Eriksen, MP; Pirkle, JL; Maurer, KR (1998). Racial and ethnic differences in serum cotinine levels of cigarette smokers: Third National Health and Nutrition Examination Survey, 1988-1991 [see comments]. *JAMA* 280 (2, 8 Jul), 135-139. [NHANES III; serum creatinine; smoking] CONTEXT: Cotinine, a metabolite of nicotine, is a marker of exposure to tobacco smoke. Previous studies suggest that non-Hispanic blacks have higher levels of serum cotinine than non-Hispanic whites who report similar levels of cigarette smoking. OBJECTIVE: To investigate differences in levels of serum cotinine in black, white, and Mexican American cigarette smokers in the US adult population. DESIGN: Third National Health and Nutrition Examination Survey, 1988-1991. PARTICIPANTS: A nationally representative sample of persons aged 17 years or older who participated in the survey. OUTCOME MEASURES: Serum cotinine levels by reported number of cigarettes smoked per day and by race and ethnicity. RESULTS: A total of 7182 subjects were involved in the study; 2136 subjects reported smoking at least 1 cigarette in the last 5 days. Black smokers had cotinine concentrations substantially higher at all levels of cigarette smoking than did white or Mexican American smokers (p<.001). Serum cotinine levels for blacks were 125 nmol/L (22 ng/mL) (95% confidence interval [CI], 79-176 nmol/L [14-31 ng/mL]) to 539 nmol/L (95 ng/mL) (95% CI, 289-630 nmol/L [51-111 ng/mL]) higher than for whites and 136 nmol/L (24 ng/mL) (95% CI, 85-182 nmol/L [15-32 ng/mL]) to 641 nmol/L (113 ng/mL) (95% CI, 386-897 nmol/L [68-158 ng/mL]) higher than for Mexican Americans. These differences do not appear to be attributable to differences in environmental tobacco smoke exposure or in number of cigarettes smoked. CONCLUSIONS: To our knowledge, this study provides the first evidence from a national study that serum cotinine levels are higher among black smokers than among white or Mexican American smokers. If higher cotinine levels among blacks indicate higher nicotine intake or differential pharmacokinetics and possibly serve as a marker of higher exposure to cigarette carcinogenic components, they may help explain why blacks find it harder to quit and are more likely to experience higher rates of lung cancer than white smokers.

Carter, CL; Jones, DY; Schatzkin, A; Brinton, LA (1989). A prospective study of reproductive, familial and socioeconomic risk factors for breast cancer using NHANES I data. *Pub.Hlth.Rep.* 104(1, Jan-Feb), 45-50. [adult; aged; breast neoplasms, epidemiology; breast neoplasms, etiology; cross-sectional studies; educational status; menarche; menopause; middle age; NHANES-I; prospective studies; risk-factors; socioeconomic factors; United States]

Carter-Pokras, O; Pirkle, J; Chavez, G; Gunter, E (1990). Blood lead levels of 4-11-year-old Mexican American, Puerto Rican, and Cuban children. *Pub. Hlth. Rep.* 105(4, Jul-Aug), 388-393. [child; child, preschool; HHANES; Hispanic Americans; lead, blood]

Carter-Pokras, OD; Gergen, PJ (1993). Reported asthma among Puerto Rican, Mexican-American, and Cuban children, 1982 through 1984. *Am. J. Pub. Hlth.* 83(4, Apr), 580-582. [absenteeism; activities of daily living; age factors; asthma, epidemiology; HHANES; Hispanic Americans, statistical and numerical data; Mexican Americans, statistical and numerical data; NHANES II; DHES].

Casty, F; Arrighi, HM (1994). Asthma and adult height attained - data from NHANES II. *J. Allergy Clin. Immunol.* 93 (1), 246. [NHANES II].

CDC (1997a). Update: blood lead levels--United States, 1991-1994 [published erratum appears in MMWR Morb Mortal Wkly Rep 1997 Jul 4;46(26):607]. *MMWR* 46, 141-146. [blood lead levels; NHANES III]
Lead is an environmental toxicant that may deleteriously affect the nervous, hematopoietic, endocrine, renal, and reproductive systems. Lead exposure in young children is a particular hazard because children absorb lead more readily than do adults and because the developing nervous systems of children are more susceptible to the effects of lead. Blood lead levels (BLLs) at least as low as 10 micrograms/dL can adversely affect the behavior and development of

children. CDC's National Health and Nutrition Examination surveys (NHANES), an ongoing series of national examinations of the health and nutritional status of the civilian noninstitutionalized population, have been the primary source for monitoring BLLs in the U.S. population. From NHANES II (conducted during 1976-1980) to Phase 1 of NHANES III (conducted during October 1988-September 1991), the geometric mean (GM) BLL for persons aged 1-74 years declined from 12.8 micrograms/dL, and the prevalence of elevated BLLs (BLLs > or = 10 micrograms/dL) decreased from 77.8% to 4.4%. This report updates national BLL estimated with data from Phase 2 of NHANES III (conducted during October 1991-September 1994), which indicate that BLLs in the U.S. population aged > or = 1 year continued to decrease and that BLLs among children aged 1-5 years were more likely to be elevated among those who were poor, non-Hispanic black, living in large metropolitan areas, or living in older housing.

CDC (1997b). Update: Blood lead levels - United States, 1991-1994 (Reprinted from MMWR, vol 46, pg 141-146, 1997). *JAMA* 277, 1031-1032. [blood lead levels; NHANES].

CDC (1997c). Use of unvented residential heating appliances--United States, 1988-1994. *MMWR* 46, 1221-1224. [heating; NHANES III].
Many heating appliances rely on combustion of carbon-based fuels and therefore are potential sources of health-threatening indoor air pollution. Most combustion heating appliances are vented to the outside of buildings to facilitate removal of the products of combustion, which include carbon monoxide (CO), carbon dioxide, nitrogen dioxide, and water vapor. However, some combustion heating devices may be unvented (e.g., kerosene- and propane-fueled space heaters, some gas-fueled log sets, and cooking devices used improperly for heating), and the use of such unvented devices in closed settings may be associated with risks for exposure to toxic gases and other emissions. This report presents an analysis of data from the Third National Health and Nutrition Examination Survey (NHANES III) to estimate the number and regional distribution of adults using unvented residential heating appliances and stoves or ovens misused as heating devices in the United States during 1988-1994. The findings indicate that the percentage of adults using these devices was higher in the South, among low-income groups, among blacks, and among rural residents, and underscore the need for public education about the health risks associated with exposure to elevated levels of combustion by-products. NHANES III collected data from approximately 20,000 adults about household characteristics, including the prevalence of various types of residential heating appliances, the use of unvented combustion space heaters, and use of stoves or ovens specifically for heating during the previous year. NHANES weights were used to obtain national estimates based on these responses. Because responses by race/ethnicity other than for whites and blacks were too small for reliable estimates, responses from all others were combined.

Centers for Disease Control and Prevention (1993): Preliminary data: exposure of persons aged > or = 4 years to tobacco smoke--United States, 1988-91. *MMWR* 42(2, Jan 22), 37-39. [adolescence; adult; aged; aged, 80 and over; child; child, preschool; cotinine, blood; middle age; NHANES-III; population surveillance; tobacco smoke pollution, analysis; DHES].

Centers for Disease Control and Prevention (1994). Blood lead levels--United States, 1988-

1991. *MMWR* 43(30, Aug 5), 545-548. [adolescence; adult; aged; child; child, preschool; lead poisoning, epidemiology; lead, blood; NHANES-III; population surveillance; DHES].

Chestnut, LG; Schwartz, J; Savitz, DA; Burchfiel, CM (1991). Pulmonary function and ambient particulate matter: epidemiological evidence from NHANES I. *Arch. Env. Hlth.* 46(3, May-Jun), 135-144. [adult; aged; air pollutants, environmental, adverse effects; air pollutants, environmental, analysis; anthropometry; forced expiratory volume; health status indicators; health surveys; maximum permissible exposure level; middle age; NHANES-I; predictive value of tests; regression analysis; respiratory tract diseases, epidemiology; respiratory tract diseases, physiopathology; socioeconomic factors; United States, epidemiology; vital capacity].

Coate, D; Grossman, M (1988). Carbon monoxide in the ambient air and blood pressure evidence from NHANES II and the SAROAD system. National Bureau of Economic Research, Cambridge, MA (1050 Massachusetts Avenue, Cambridge, Mass. 02138). [NHANES II]

Coate, D; Fowles, R (1989). Is there statistical evidence for a blood lead-blood pressure relationship? *J. Health Econ.* 8(2), 173-184. [blood pressure; hypertension, epidemiology; lead blood level; NHANES-II; statistical analysis; United States].

Cohen, BB; Friedman, DJ; Mahan, CM; Lederman, R; Munoz, D (1993). Ethnicity, maternal risk, and birth-weight among Hispanics in Massachusetts, 1987-89. *Pub. Hlth. Rep.* 108(3), 363-371. [HHANES].

Collins, JW; Shay, DK (1994). Prevalence of low-birth-weight among Hispanic infants with United States-born and foreign-born mothers -the effect of urban poverty. *Am. J. Epid.* 139 (2),184-192. [acculturation; birth weight; Black; depressive symptoms; health; HHANES 1982-84; Hispanic Americans; Mexican-American population; mortality; poverty]

Cooper, RS; Ford, E (1992). Comparability of risk factors for coronary heart disease among blacks and whites in the NHANES-I Epidemiologic Follow-up Study. *Ann. Epid.* 2(5), 637-645. [adult; African-American; body mass; caucasian; cholesterol, endogenous compound; coronary risk; female; follow-up; hospitalization; human; incidence; ischemic heart disease, epidemiology; life style; major clinical study; male; mortality; NHANES-I; NHEFS; race difference; smoking; systolic blood pressure; United States]

Cowie CC; Harris MI; Silverman RE; Johnson EW; Rust KF (1993): Effect of multiple risk factors on differences between blacks and whites in the prevalence of non-insulin-dependent diabetes mellitus in the United States. Am. J. Epidemiol. 137(7, Apr 1), 719-732. [BLACKS; DIABETES MELLITUS, NON-INSULIN-DEPENDENT, ETHNOLOGY; NHANES II].

Crocetti, AF; Mushak, P; Schwartz, J (1990). Determination of numbers of lead-exposed women of childbearing age and pregnant women: an integrated summary of a report to the U.S. Congress on childhood lead poisoning. *Env. Hlth. Persp.* 89(Nov), 121-124. [adolescence; adult; epidemiologic methods; fetus, drug effects; lead poisoning, blood; lead poisoning, complications; lead poisoning, epidemiology; lead, blood; NHANES-II; pregnancy complications, epidemiology].

DeBaun, MR; Sox, HC Jr (1991). Setting the optimal erythrocyte protoporphyrin screening decision threshold for lead poisoning: a decision analytic approach. *Pediatrics* 88(1, Jul), 121-131. [child; decision support techniques; erythrocytes, chemistry; lead poisoning, diagnosis; NHANES-II; protoporphyrin, blood].

Dreon, DM; John, EM; DiCiccio, Y; Whittemore, AS (1993). Use of NHANES data to assign nutrient densities to food groups in a multiethnic diet history questionnaire. *Nutrition and Cancer*
20(3), 223-230. [adult; aged; data interpretation, statistical; diet surveys; food analysis; middle age; NHANES-II; nutrition assessment; Whites].

Eck, LH; Hackett-Renner, C; Klesges, LM (1992). Impact of diabetic status, dietary intake, physical activity, and smoking status on body mass index in NHANES II. *Clin. Nutr.* 56(2, Aug), 329-333. [body mass index; diabetes mellitus, non-insulin-dependent, metabolism; eating, physiology; NHANES II].

Engel, A; Johnson, ML; Haynes, SG (1988). Health effects of sunlight exposure in the United States. Results from the first National Health and Nutrition Examination Survey, 1971-1974. *Arch. Dermatol.* 124(1, Jan), 72-79. [NHANES I; skin diseases, epidemiology; sunlight, adverse effects].

Enstrom, JE. (1999). Smoking cessation and mortality trends among two United States populations. *J. Clin. Epidemiol.* 52 (9, Sep), 813-825. [mortality; NHEFS; smoking].
The long-term impact of smoking cessation on mortality is assessed among two U.S. populations: a large cohort of U.S. veterans aged 55-64 at entry and followed from 1954 through 1979 and the NHANES I Epidemiologic Followup Study (NHEFS) cohort of a national sample of U.S. adults aged 55-74 at entry and followed from 1971 through 1992. Direct and indirect survey data indicate that 50-70% of those who were current cigarette smokers at entry had quit smoking during the 19- to 26- year follow-up periods. The impact of smoking cessation on mortality among the cigarette smokers as a whole has been assessed by determining the time trend of the relative risk (RR) of death and 95% confidence interval (CI) for the cigarette smokers compared with never-smokers over the entire follow-up period in both cohorts. The total death rates for the 1954/57 U.S. veteran smokers as a whole (63,159 males) have converged only slightly toward those of never-smokers, from RR = 1.65 (1.58-1.72) during 1954-1959 to RR = 1.61 (1.58-1.63) during 1954-1979. The lung cancer death rates for 1954/57 smokers as a whole have not converged toward those of never-smokers, with RR = 10.89 (7.70-15.41) during 1954-1959 and RR = 11.10 (9.78-12.61) during 1954-1979. The total death rates for the 1971-1975 NHEFS smokers as a whole (694 males and 1116 females) have not converged toward those
of never-smokers. For males, RR = 1.92 (1.46-2.52) during 1971-1982 and RR = 1.96 (1.63-2.36) during 1971-1992; for females, RR = 1.79 (1.31-2.46) during 1971-1982 and RR = 1.79

(1.47-2.17) during 1971- 1992. The lung cancer death rates have diverged, based on small numbers of deaths. For males, RR = 15.76 (2.06-120.61) during 1971-1982 and RR = 22.20 (5.31-92.92) during 1971-1992; for females, RR = 2.92 (0.57-15.06) during 1971-1982 and RR = 4.74 (1.94-11.59) during 1971-1992. These trends are contrary to the substantial convergence predicted by the death rate trends among U.S. veterans who were former smokers at the beginning of follow-up. While these results confirm that those former smokers who survive for at least 5 years experience death rates that converge toward those of never-smokers, they also indicate that a cohort of cigarette smokers that undergoes substantial cessation experiences a death rate that does not converge toward the death rate of never-smokers. The fact that there has been no convergence for lung cancer is quite surprising, as this is the disease most strongly linked to smoking and smoking cessation and less likely to be influenced by other lifestyle factors. Further investigation is needed for a complete understanding of the impact of smoking cessation.

Escobedo, LG; Remington, PL (1989). Birth cohort analysis of prevalence of cigarette smoking among Hispanics in the United States. *JAMA* 261(1, Jan 6), 66-69. [adolescence; adult; aged; cohort studies; Cuba, ethnology; HHANES; Hispanic Americans, psychology; smoking, ethnology]

Escobedo, LG; Remington, PL; Anda, RF (1989). Long-term age-specific prevalence of cigarette smoking among Hispanics in the United States. *J. Psychoactive Drugs* 21(3, Jul-Sep), 307-318.
[adolescence; adult; age factors; aged; Cuba, ethnology; HHANES; Hispanic Americans, psychology; smoking, epidemiology]

Escobedo, LG; Remington, PL; Anda, RF (1989). Long-term secular trends in initiation of cigarette smoking among Hispanics in the United States. *Pub. Hlth. Rep.* 104(6, Nov-Dec), 583-587. [adult; HHANES; Hispanic Americans; smoking, ethnology]

Espino, DV; Moreno, C; Katerndahl, D; Wood, R (1990). Serum lead and hypertension in older Mexican-Americans - the HHANES. *J. Am. Geriatr. Soc.* 38(8), 16. [HHANES; hypertension; serum lead].

Ezzati-Rice, TM; Murphy, RS (1995). Issues associated with the design of a national probability sample for human exposure assessment. *Env. Hlth. Persp.* 103 Suppl 3(Apr), 55-59.
[data collection; environmental exposure; epidemiologic methods; Hazardous substances; national health programs; NHANES III; Probability; research design; risk assessment; DHES].

Fanelli-Kuczmarski, MT; Johnson, CL; Elias, L; Najjar, MF (1990). Folate status of Mexican American, Cuban, and Puerto Rican women. *Am. J. Clin. Nutr.* 52(2, Aug), 368-372. [adult; cuba, ethnology; educational status; erythrocytes, analysis; folic acid, blood; HHANES; Hispanic Americans; DHES].

Farfel, M (1987). Evaluation of health and environmental effects of two methods for residential lead paint removal. SC.D Thesis, The Johns Hopkins University, 315 p. [health sciences, public health; NHANES-II; thesis].

Flegal, KM (1990). Ratio of actual to predicted weight as an alternative to a power-type weight-height index (Benn index). *Clin. Nutr.* 51(4, Apr), 540-547. [adult; age factors; body height; body mass index; body weight; NHANES II; DHES]

Frisancho, AR; Ryan, AS (1991). Decreased stature associated with moderate blood lead concentrations in Mexican-American children. *Clin. Nutr.* 54(3, Sep), 516-519. [age factors; body height; HHANES; Hispanic Americans; lead, blood]

Garg, R; Madams, JH; Kleinman, JC (1992). Regional variation in ischemic heart disease incidence. *J. Clin. Epid.* 45(2, Feb), 149-156. [aged; body mass index; coronary disease, epidemiology; coronary disease, mortality; diabetes mellitus, complications; educational status; follow-up studies; NHANES-I; NHEFS; residence characteristics]

Gartside, PS (1988). The relationship of blood lead levels and blood pressure in NHANES II: additional calculations. *Env. Hlth. Persp.* 78(Jun), 31-34. [adult; aged; blood pressure, drug effects; lead, blood; NHANES II].

Gartside, PS; Wang, P; Glueck CJ (1998a). Prospective assessment of cancer morbidity/mortality risk factors: The NHANES I 16 year Epidemiologic Followup Study - meeting abstract. *J. Investig. Med.* 46 (N3, Mar), A212-A212. [cancer; CHD; NHANES I; NHEFS].

Gartside, PS; Glueck, CJ (1993). Relationship of dietary intake to hospital admission for coronary heart and vascular disease: the NHANES II National Probability Study. *J. Am. Coll. Nutr.* 12(6, Dec), 676-684. [alcohol drinking; caffeine; cholesterol, blood; coronary disease; diet; hospitalization; NHANES-II; nutrition; vascular diseases].

Gartside, PS; Glueck, CJ (1994). Inverse association of milk intake with cancer morbidity and mortality, the prospective NHANES I Epidemiologic Follow-up-study. *Clin. Res.* 42(3), A380. [NHANES I; NHEFS]

Gergen, PJ; Mullally, DI; Evans, R 3d (1988). National survey of prevalence of asthma among children in the United States, 1976 to 1980. *Pediatrics* 81(1, Jan), 1-7. [adolescence; asthma, diagnosis; asthma, epidemiology; asthma, immunology; child; NHANES-II; skin tests; United States; DHES]

Gergen, PJ; Turkeltaub, PC (1988). The association of percutaneous immediate hypersensitivity and respiratory symptoms in the United States population - data from the second National Health and Nutrition Examination Survey - 1976-80 (NHANES-II). *J. Allergy Clin. Immunol.* 81(1), 174. [NHANES II; DHES]

Gergen, PJ; Weiss, KB (1990). Changing patterns of asthma hospitalization among United States children 0-17 years of age: 1979-87. *JAMA* 264, 1688-1692. [NHANES II; DHES]

Gergen, PJ; Turkeltaub, PC (1991). The association of allergen skin test reactivity and respiratory disease among whites in the US population. Data from the second National Health and Nutrition Examination Survey, 1976 to 1980. *Arch. Intern. Med.* 151(3, Mar), 487-492. [adolescence; adult; aged; child; cross-sectional studies; health surveys; middle age; NHANES-II; nutrition surveys; prevalence; regression analysis; respiratory hypersensitivity, epidemiology; sampling studies; skin tests; United States, epidemiology; DHES]

Gergen, PJ; Turkeltaub, PC (1992). The association of individual allergen reactivity with respiratory disease in a national sample: data from the second National Health and Nutrition Examination Survey, 1976-80 (NHANES II). *J. Allergy Clin.Immunol.* 90(4 Pt 1, Oct), 579-588. [adolescence; adult; allergens, immunology; health surveys; NHANES-II; respiratory hypersensitivity, immunology; DHES]

Gergen, PJ; Turkeltaub, PC; Kramer, RA (1992). Age of onset in childhood asthma: data from a national cohort. *Ann. Allergy* 68(6, Jun), 507-514. [adolescence; adult; age factors; asthma, etiology; NHANES II; DHES]

Gergen, PJ; Fowler, JA; Maurer, KR; Davis, WW; Overpeck, MD (1998). The burden of environmental tobacco smoke exposure on the respiratory health of children 2 months through 5 years of age in the United States: third National Health and Nutrition Examination Survey, 1988 to 1994. Pediatrics 101 (2, Feb), E8. [asthma; children; NHANES-III; smoking; tobacco] OBJECTIVE: To measure the effect of environmental tobacco smoke (ETS) on respiratory health in a national sample of young children. METHODS: The study evaluated children 2 months through 5 years of age participating in the Third National Health and Nutrition Examination Survey, 1988 to 1994. The group was a representative sample of the US population (N = 7680). A parental report of household smoking or maternal smoking during pregnancy ascertained ETS exposure. Respiratory outcomes were based on parental report of wheezing, cough, upper respiratory infection, or pneumonia in the last 12 months and chronic bronchitis or physician-diagnosed asthma at any time. Logistic regression was used to adjust for age, sex, race/ethnicity, birth weight, day care, family history of allergy, breast-feeding, education level of head of household, and household size. RESULTS: Approximately 38% of children were presently exposed to ETS in the home, whereas 23.8% were exposed by maternal smoking during pregnancy. ETS exposure increased chronic bronchitis and three or more episodes of wheezing
among children 2 months to 2 years old and asthma among children 2 months to 5 years old. For household exposure, a consistent effect was seen only at >/=20 cigarettes smoked per day. Adjusted odds ratios for increased risk (95% confidence interval) for household exposures (>/=20 cigarettes smoked per day vs none smoked) and maternal prenatal exposure (prenatal smoking vs no smoking), respectively, for children 2 months to 2 years old were chronic bronchitis, 2.5 (1.6, 4.1); 2.2, (1.6, 3); three or more episodes of wheezing, 2.7 (1.7, 4.2), 2.1 (1. 5, 2.9); and for children 2 months to 5 years old were asthma, 2.1 (1.4, 3.2); 1.8 (1.3, 2.6).

Reported use within the past month of prescription medications for asthma (beta-agonists or inhaled steroids) was not different between those with asthma reporting ETS exposure and those reporting no exposure; percent of patients with asthma reporting use of medication by household exposure was 0, 25. 7%; 1 to 19 cigarettes smoked per day, 32.9%; and >/=20 cigarettes smoked per day, 23.1%; percent of patients with asthma reporting use of medication by maternal smoking during pregnancy was no, 28.9%; yes, 22.7%. Among children 2 months to 2 years of age exposed to ETS, 40% to 60% of the cases of asthma, chronic bronchitis, and three or more episodes of wheezing were attributable to ETS exposure. For diagnosed asthma among children 2 months through 5 years old, there were 133 800 to 161 600 excess cases. Among exposed children 2 months through 2 years of age, there were 61 000 to 79 200 excess cases of chronic bronchitis and 126 700 to 172 000 excess cases of three or more episodes of wheezing. CONCLUSIONS: ETS exposure is common among children in the United States. The reported prevalence of asthma, wheezing, and chronic bronchitis was increased with ETS exposures. No statistically significant increase in the prevalence of upper respiratory infection, pneumonia, or cough was associated with ETS exposure. ETS exposure has little effect on the respiratory health of children between 3 and 5 years of age, with the exception of asthma. ETS appears to increase the prevalence of asthma rather than the severity as measured by medication use. These findings reinforce the need to reduce the exposure of young children to ETS.

Geronimus, AT; Hillemeier, MM (1992). Patterns of blood lead levels in US black and white women of childbearing age. *Ethn. Dis.* 2(3,Summer), 222-231. [adolescence; adult; age factors; blacks, statistical and numerical data; environmental exposure; lead poisoning, epidemiology; NHANES-II; whites, statistical and numerical data]

Gottlieb, DJ; Beiser, AS; O'Connor, GT (1995). Poverty, race, and medication use are correlates of asthma hospitalization rates - a small-area analysis in Boston. *Chest* 108 (1), 28-35. [asthma; changing patterns; childhood asthma; children; epidemiology; exposure; health; particulate air-pollution; medication; NHANES; poverty; risk-factors; small-area analysis; smoking; United States].

Goyer, RA (1990). Lead toxicity: from overt to subclinical to subtle health effects. *Env. Hlth. Persp.* 86(Jun), 177-181. [behavior, drug effects; lead, adverse effects; NHANES II]

Guendelman, S; Abrams, B (1994). Dietary, alcohol, and tobacco intake among Mexican-American women of childbearing age: Results from HANES data. *Am. J. Health Promot.* 8(5), 363-372. [adolescent; adult; alcohol consumption; caucasian; comparison; demography; dietary intake; ethnic group; feeding behavior; female; fluid intake; health behavior; health survey; HHANES; human; lactation; major clinical study; maternal nutrition; pregnancy; prenatal period; puerperium; smoking; social status]

Hahn, RA; Eaker, E; Barker, ND; Teutsch, SM; Sosniak, W; Krieger, N (1995). Poverty and death in the United States - 1973 and 1991. *Epid.* 6(5), 490-497. [cholesterol blood level; death; health statistics; NHANES-I; poverty; risk assessment; risk factor; smoking; statistical analysis; survival]

Hankinson, JL; Odencrantz, JR; Fedan, KB (1999). Spirometric reference values from a sample of the general U.S. population. *Am. J. Respir. Crit. Care. Med.* 159 (1, Jan), 179-87. [Black Americans; Mexican Americans; NHANES-III; spirometry; White Americans]
Spirometric reference values for Caucasians, African-Americans, and Mexican-Americans 8 to 80 yr of age were developed from 7,429 asymptomatic, lifelong nonsmoking participants in the third National Health and Nutrition Examination Survey (NHANES III). Spirometry examinations followed the 1987 American Thoracic Society recommendations, and the quality of the data was continuously monitored and maintained. Caucasian subjects had higher mean FVC and FEV1 values than did Mexican-American and African-American subjects across the entire age range. However, Caucasian and Mexican-American subjects had similar FVC and FEV1 values with respect to height, and African-American subjects had lower values. These differences may be partially due to differences in body build: observed Mexican-Americans were shorter than Caucasian subjects of the same age, and African-Americans on average have a smaller trunk:leg ratio than do Caucasians. Reference values and lower limits of normal were derived using a piecewise polynomial model with age and height as predictors. These reference values encompass a wide age range for three race/ethnic groups and should prove useful for diagnostic and research purposes.

Harlan, WR (1988). The relationship of blood lead levels to blood pressure in the U.S. population. *Env. Hlth. Persp.* 78(Jun), 9-13. [adolescence; blood pressure, drug effects; lead, blood; NHANES II]

Huseman, CA; Varma, MM; Angle, CR (1992). Neuroendocrine effects of toxic and low blood lead levels in children. *Pediatrics* 90(2 Pt 1, Aug), 186-189. [Insulin-like Growth Factor I, analysis; lead, blood; NHANES II]

Istvan, JA; Cunningham, TW (1992). Smoking rate, carboxyhemoglobin, and body mass in the second National Health and Nutrition Examination Survey (NHANES II). *J. Behav. Med.* 15(6, Dec), 559-572. [body weight; carboxyhemoglobin, analysis; NHANES-II; nutrition surveys]

Istvan, JA; Nides, MA; Buist, AS; Greene, P; Voelker, H (1994). Salivary cotinine, frequency of cigarette-smoking, and body-mass index - findings at base-line in the lung health study. *Am. J. Epid.* 139(6), 628-636. [2nd National Health; body weight; cotinine; energy-expenditure; nutrition examination survey; NHANES-II; nicotine; obesity; population; smokers; smoking; weight; women]

Jenkins, RA; Counts, RW (1999). Personal exposure to environmental tobacco smoke: salivary cotinine, airborne nicotine, and nonsmoker misclassification. *J. Expo. Anal. Environ. Epidemiol.* 9 (4, Jul-Aug), 352-363. [cotinine; EPA; lung cancer; NHANES-III; smoking]
A large study was conducted to assess exposure to environmental tobacco smoke (ETS) in a geographically dispersed study population using personal breathing zone air sampling and salivary cotinine levels. Approximately 100 self-reported nonsmoking subjects in each of 16 metropolitan areas were recruited for this investigation. Cumulative distributions of salivary cotinine levels for subjects in smoking and nonsmoking homes and workplaces exhibited a

general trend of decreasing salivary cotinine levels with decreasing time spent in smoking environments. Median salivary cotinine levels for the four experimental cells in the study (product of smoking and nonsmoking home and workplaces) were comparable to those reported for a large national study of serum levels of cotinine (Third National Health and Nutrition Examination Survey, NHANES III), when the latter was corrected for expected differences between serum and saliva concentrations. However, the most highly exposed group in this study had a median salivary cotinine concentration approximately a factor of 2 greater than that of the comparable group in the NHANES III study. Misclassification rates, both simple (for self-reported nonsmokers) and complex (self-reported lifetime never smokers), were near the median of those reported for other studies. Estimated misclassification rates for self-reported lifetime never-smoking females are sufficiently high (2.95% using a discrimination level of 106 ng/ml) that, if used in the Environmental Protection Agency (EPA) risk assessment related to ETS and lung cancer, would place the lower 90% confidence interval (CI) for relative risk at nearly 1.00, i.e., no statistically significant increased risk. For the 263 most highly exposed subjects in the study whose self-reported nonsmoking status was accurate, the correlation between airborne exposure to nicotine and average salivary cotinine is so small, on an individual basis, that it makes the relationship useless for estimating exposure on a quantitative basis. When subjects are grouped according to likely categories of nicotine exposure, correlation between group median airborne nicotine exposure and salivary cotinine level increases dramatically. The comparison improves for the most highly exposed subjects, suggesting that such quantitative comparisons are useful for only those subjects who are exposed to the higher levels of ETS. However, airborne nicotine exposure for most of the subjects does not account for estimated systemic levels of nicotine, based on salivary cotinine levels.

John, EM; Schwartz, GG; Dreon, DM; Koo J (1999): Vitamin D and breast cancer risk: the NHANES I Epidemiologic follow-up study, 1971-1975 to 1992. National Health and Nutrition Examination Survey. *Cancer Epidemiol Biomarkers* 8 (5, May), 399-406. [breast cancer; NHEFS; Vitamin D]
We analyzed data from the first National Health and Nutrition Examination Survey Epidemiologic Follow-up Study to test the hypothesis that vitamin D from sunlight exposure, diet, and supplements reduces the risk of breast cancer. We identified 190 women with incident breast cancer from a cohort of 5009 white women who completed the dermatological examination and 24-h dietary recall conducted from1971-1974 and who were followed up to 1992. Using Cox proportional hazards regression, we estimated relative risks (RRs) for breast cancer and 95% confidence intervals, adjusting for age, education, age at menarche, age at menopause, body mass index, alcohol consumption, and physical activity. Several measures of sunlight exposure and dietary vitamin D intake were associated with reduced risk of breast cancer, with RRs ranging from 0.67-0.85. The associations with vitamin D exposures, however, varied by region of residence. The risk reductions were highest for women who lived in United States regions of high solar radiation, with RRs ranging from 0.35-0.75. No reductions in risk were found for women who lived in regions of low solar radiation. Although limited by the relatively small size of the case population, the protective effects of vitamin D observed in this prospective study are consistent for several independent measures of vitamin D. These data support the hypothesis that sunlight and dietary vitamin D reduce the risk of breast cancer.

Jones, CP (1995). Methods for comparing distributions development and application exploring "race"-associated differences in systolic blood pressure. PH.D. Thesis, The Johns Hopkins University, 356 p. [biology, biostatistics; health sciences, public health; NHANES I; NHANES II].

Jones, DY; Schatzkin, A; Green, SB; Block, G; Brinton, LA; Ziegler, RG; Hoover, R; Taylor, PR (1987). Dietary fat and breast cancer in the National Health and Nutrition Examination Survey I Epidemiologic Follow-up Study. *J. Natl. Cancer Inst.* 79(3, Sep), 465-471. [adult; age factors; aged; breast neoplasms, epidemiology; breast neoplasms, etiology; caloric intake; dietary fats, administration and dosage; dietary fats, adverse effects; follow-up studies; menarche; NHANES I; NHEFS]

Kant, AK; Schatzkin, A; Block, G; Ziegler, RG; Nestle, M (1991). Food group intake patterns and associated nutrient profiles of the US population. *J. Am. Diet. Assoc.* 91(12, Dec), 1532-1537. [adult; aged; anthropometry; ascorbic acid, blood; blacks; diet; diet records; diet surveys; eating; food preferences; middle age; NHANES-II; nutrition; United States; whites].

Kennedy, A (1987). Serum cholesterol and cancer in the NHANES I Epidemiological Follow up Study [letter]. *Lancet* 2(8567, Nov 7), 1096. [adult; cholesterol, blood; neoplasms, epidemiology; NHANES I; NHEFS]

Kimmel, CA; Neumann, DA (1997). Accounting for susceptibility in risk assessment: Current practice and new directions. *Env. Tox. and Pharm.* 4, 189-194. [chemical exposures; NHANES; risk assessments]

Differences in susceptibility between individuals can lead to variability in response to chemical exposures which in turn modify the risk of illness. As a means of exploring the basis for such differences in susceptibility, a project was undertaken to determine what data were available on the range of response variability for several health effects: neurotoxicity, reproductive/developmental toxicity, pulmonary toxicity, and cancer. In addition, modeling approaches for characterizing response variability were examined and evaluated. The main goal of this effort was to determine whether human response variability was adequately accounted for in the current risk assessment procedures for human health effects. The conclusions of the project were that few data are available, both because variability has rarely been the primary focus of study, and because data are not usually reported in such a way that response variability can be determined. Several recommendations were made to facilitate better characterization of interindividual variability, including the study of variability in available human data (e.g. the NHANES database) and allowing greater access to raw data from epidemiologic studies. In addition, the identification of relevant biomarkers, improved understanding of sources of variability, interaction of chemical effects with other exposures or pre-existing disease, and retrospective evaluations of risk assessments were recommended. It is hoped that these recommendations will stimulate research on susceptibility and response variability and encourage the reporting of data in a way that facilitates analysis of interindividual variability in response.

Klein, BE; Cruickshanks, KJ; Klein, R (1995). Leisure time, sunlight exposure and cataracts. *Doc. Ophthalmol.* 88(3-4), 295-305. [adult; aged; cataract, epidemiology; cataract, etiology; environmental exposure, adverse effects; leisure activities; lens, crystalline, radiation effects; middle age; NHANES-I; radiation injuries, epidemiology; radiation injuries, etiology; risk-factors; sunlight, adverse effects; time factors]

Klein, R; Rowland, ML; Harris, MI (1995). Racial/ethnic differences in age-related maculopathy. Third National Health and Nutrition Examination Survey. *Ophthalmology* 102(3, Mar), 371-381.
[adult; aged; aged, 80 and over; caucasoid race; ethnic groups, statistical and numerical data; macula lutea, pathology; macular degeneration, ethnology; macular degeneration, pathology; Mexican-Americans; middle age; negroid race; NHANES-III; photography; prevalence; racial stocks; United States, epidemiology; DHES]

Klesges, RC; Klesges, LM; Meyers, AW (1991). Relationship of smoking status, energy balance, and body weight: analysis of the second National Health and Nutrition Examination Survey. *J. Consult.Clin. Psychol.* 59(6, Dec), 899-905. [body weight, physiology; energy metabolism, physiology; NHANES II]

Klesges, RC; Eck, LH; Ray, JW (1995). Who under reports dietary intake in a dietary recall? Evidence from the second National Health and Nutrition Examination Survey. *J. Consult. Clin. Psychol.* 63(3, Jun), 438-444. [caloric intake; NHANES-II; nutrition surveys; recall; truth disclosure].

Kowal, NE (1988). Urinary cadmium and beta 2-microglobulin: correlation with nutrition and smoking history. *J. Tox. Env. Hlth.* 25(2), 179-183. [beta 2-microglobulin, urine; cadmium, urine; NHANES II]

Kritchevsky, SB (1992). Dietary lipids and the low blood cholesterol-cancer association. *Am. J. Epid.* 135(5, Mar 1), 509-520. [age factors; cholesterol, blood; diet surveys; dietary fats, administration and dosage; follow-up studies; interviews; logistic models; neoplasms, epidemiology; NHANES I; NHEFS]

Kurtin, D; Therrell, BL Jr; Patterson, P (1997). Demographic risk factors associated with elevated lead levels in Texas children covered by Medicaid. *Env. Hlth. Persp.* 105, 66-68. [lead levels; NHANES II; NHANES III]
This is the first large population-based study of demographic risk factors for elevated lead in Texas children. It summarizes data on 92,900 children covered by Medicaid screened for blood lead during the first 6 months of 1993 in Texas. The highest percentage of elevated lead levels (14.3%) was in children 25-36 months of age, with slightly lower percentages in those younger (13% of 19-24 months) and older (12% of 37-48 months) with blood lead levels greater than 10 micrograms/dl. The group with the highest percentage of elevated blood lead levels was 2-4-year-old African American males (17.3%) making this subgroup 3.5 times higher than the group with the lowest percentage-white girls over age 4 (4.8%). Males had higher blood lead levels for

all ages and ethnic groups. Three principal risk factors were found for excessive blood lead in children: ethnicity, gender, and age; this is consistent with the second National Health and Nutrition Examination Survey (NHANES II) and Phase I of the NHANES III results demonstrating ethnicity and income association with lead in children in the United States.

Kutz, FW; Cook, BT; Carter-Pokras, OD; Brody, DJ; Murphy, RS (1992). Selected pesticide residues and metabolites in urine from a survey of the U.S. general population. *J. Tox. Env. Hlth.* 37(2, Oct), 277-291. [adolescence; adult; age factors; aged; chlorophenols, urine; NHANES-II, pentachlorophenol, urine; pesticide residues, urine; DHES].

Landis, JR; Flegal, KM (1988). A generalized Mantel-Haenszel analysis of the regression of blood pressure on blood lead using NHANES II data. *Env. Hlth. Persp.* 78(Jun), 35-41. [adolescence; blood pressure, drug effects; lead, blood; NHANES II; DHES]

Lee, DJ; Markides, KS (1991). Health behaviors, risk factors, and health indicators associated with cigarette use in Mexican Americans: results from the Hispanic HANES. *Am. J. Pub. Hlth.* 81(7, Jul), 859-864. [activities of daily living; adult; aged; alcohol drinking, epidemiology; health behavior; health status indicators; HHANES; Hispanic Americans, psychology; smoking, ethnology]

Leidy, L (1998): Menarche, menopause, and migration: Implications for breast cancer research. *Am. J. Human Biology* 10 (N4), 451-457. [cancer; HHANES; menarche; menopause]
A multi generational delay in the rise of breast cancer incidence rates has been documented among immigrants to the United States. Prompted by this observation, this study examines three breast cancer risk factors, age at menarche, parity, and age at menopause, in relation to each other and in relation to migration status and language most often used in U.S. Hispanic populations. Mexican American (n = 1,502), Cuban American (n = 534), and Puerto Rican(n = 700) women, aged 30-74 years, were drawn from the Hispanic Health and Nutrition Examination Survey (HHANES), 1982-1984. Mean recalled age at menarche was significantly later among first generation compared to second generation immigrants in both Mexican Americans (13.3 vs 12.8 years) and Puerto Ricans (12.8 vs 11.9 years). Among Mexican Americans, more children were reported by first generation immigrants than women of the third or more generations (4.9 vs 4.0 children) and by Spanish speakers compared to women who used English more frequently (4.5 vs 3.3 children). Mean and median ages at menopause were later among second generation Mexican American women than first generation women. There was a small, significant, positive correlation between recalled ages at menarche and menopause within each of the first generation Hispanic subgroups. The unique positive correlation between ages at menarche and menopause among first generation immigrants may relate to having spent early years in the country of origin and later years in the United States.

Leske, MC; Chylack, LT; Wu, SY (1991). The lens opacities case-control study - risk-factors for cataract. *Arch. Ophthalmol.* 109(2), 244-251. [allopurinol therapy; american diet; classification-system; NHANES-II; nuclear; nutrient sources; population; quantitative data; senile cataract; sunlight]

Linn, S; Fulwood, R; Carroll, M; Brook, JG; Johnson, C; Kalsbeek, WD; Rifkind, BM (1991). Serum total cholesterol: HDL cholesterol ratios in US white and black adults by selected demographic and socioeconomic variables (HANES II). *Am. J. Pub. Hlth.* 81(8, Aug), 1038-1043. [adult; aged; alcohol drinking; body mass index; cholesterol, blood; Framingham study; lipoproteins, hdl cholesterol, blood; negroid race; NHANES II; DHES]

Madans, JH; Reuben, CA; Rothwell, ST; Eberhardt, MS (1995). Differences in morbidity measures and risk factor identification using multiple data sources: the case of coronary heart disease [see comments]. *Stat. Med.* 14(5-7, Mar 15-Apr 15), 643-653. [aged; algorithms; coronary disease, epidemiology; databases, factual; death certificates; epidemiologic methods; follow-up studies; health surveys; incidence; middle age; models, statistical; NHANES-I; regression analysis; risk assessment; risk-factors; sex distribution; United States, epidemiology]

Madigan, MP; Ziegler, RG; Benichou, J; Byrne, C; Hoover, RN (1995). Proportion of breast cancer cases in the United States explained by well-established risk factors. *J. Natl. Cancer Inst.* 87(22, Nov 15), 1681-1685. [adult; age factors; aged; breast neoplasms, epidemiology; breast neoplasms, etiology; breast neoplasms, genetics; income; middle age; NHNAES-I; NHEFS; parity; pregnancy]

Mannino, DM; Petty, TL (1998). Obstructive lung diseases and low lung function in the United States population, 1988-94: Results from NHANES III - meeting abstract. *Am. J. Epid.* 147 (N11,S, 1 Jun), 53-53. (111 Market Place, Ste 840, Baltimore, MD 21202-6709) [lung diseases; NHANES III].

Marcus, AH; Schwartz, J (1987). Dose-response curves for erythrocyte protoporphyrin vs blood lead: effects of iron status. *Env. Res.* 44(2, Dec), 221-227. [erythrocytes, metabolism; iron, deficiency; NHANES II]

Marks, G; Garcia, M; Solis, JM (1990). Health risk behaviors of Hispanics in the United States: Findings from HHANES, 1982-84. *Am. J. Pub. Hlth.* 80(Suppl), 20-26. [adult; aged; alcohol; cigarette smoking; diet; ethnic group; female; health behavior; HHANES; human; male; mass screening; normal human; risk]

Matanoski, G; Kanchanaraksa, S; Lantry, D; Chang, Y (1995). Characteristics of nonsmoking women in NHANES I and NHANES I Epidemiologic Follow-up Study with exposure to spouses who smoke. *Am. J. Epid.* 142(2, Jul 15), 149-157. [adult; follow-up studies; NHANES I; NHEFS; nutrition; tobacco smoke pollution].

McWhorter, WP (1988). Allergy and risk of cancer. A prospective study using NHANES I follow-up data. *Cancer* 62(2, Jul 15), 451-455. [adult; aged; follow-up studies; hypersensitivity, complications; middle age; neoplasms, epidemiology; NHANES-I; NHEFS; prospective studies]

McWhorter, WP; Polis, MA; Kaslow, RA (1989). Occurrence, predictors, and consequences of adult asthma in NHANES I and Follow-up Survey. *Am. Rev. Respir. Dis.* 139(3, Mar), 721-724.

[adult; aged; aged, 80 and over; asthma, epidemiology; NHANES I; NHEFS]

Morabia, A; Sorenson, A; Kumanyika, SK; Abbey, H; Cohen, BH; Chee, E (1989). Vitamin A, cigarette smoking, and airway obstruction. *Am. Rev. Respir. Dis.* 140(5, Nov), 1312-1316. [adult; airway obstruction; NHANES-I; smoking; Vitamin A, pharmacology]

Nash, D; Silbergeld, E; Magder, L; Stolley, P (1998). Menopause, hormone replacement therapy (HRT), and blood lead levels among adult women from NHANES III, 1988-1994 - abstract. *Am. J. Epid.* 147 (N11,S, 1 Jun), L7-L7. [blood lead levels; NHANES III].

Neas, LM; Schwartz, J (1998a): Pulmonary function levels as predictors of mortality in a national sample of US adults. *Am. J. Epid.* 147 (11, 1 Jun), 1011-1018. [mortality; NHANES-I; pulmonary function]
Single breath pulmonary diffusing capacity for carbon monoxide (DL(CO)) was examined as a predictor of all-cause mortality among 4,333 subjects who were aged 25-74 years at baseline in the First National Health and Nutrition Examination Survey (NHANES I) conducted from 1971 to 1975. The relation of the percentage of predicted DL(CO) to all-cause mortality was examined in a Cox proportional hazard model that included age, sex, race, current smoking status, systolic blood pressure, serum cholesterol, alcohol consumption, body mass index, percentage of predicted forced vital capacity (FVC), and the ratio of forced expiratory volume at 1 second (FEV1) to FVC. Mortality had a linear association with the percentage of predicted FVC (rate ratio (RR) = 1.12, 95% confidence interval (CI) 1.08-1.17, for a 10% decrement) and a significantly nonlinear association with the percentage of predicted DL(CO) with an adverse effect that was clearly evident for levels below 85% of those predicted (RR = 1.24, 95% CI 1.12-1.37 for a 10% decrement). The relative hazard for the percentage of predicted DL(CO) below 85% was not modified by sex, smoking status, or exclusion of subjects with clinical respiratory disease on the initial examination. This association with the percentage of predicted DL(CO) was present among 3,005 subjects with FEV1 levels above 90% of those predicted. Thus, pulmonary diffusing capacity below 85% of predicted levels is a significant predictor of the all-cause mortality rate within the general US population independent of standard spirometry measures and even in the absence of apparent clinical respiratory disease.

Neas, LM; Schwartz, J (1998b). Pulmonary function levels as predictors of mortality in a national sample of US adults. Am J Epidemiol 147 (11, 1 Jun), 1011-1118. [alcohol; BMI; cholesterol; mortality; NHANES-I; pulmonary function; smoking; systolic blood pressure]
Single breath pulmonary diffusing capacity for carbon monoxide (DL(CO)) was examined as a predictor of all-cause mortality among 4,333 subjects who were aged 25-74 years at baseline in the First National Health and Nutrition Examination Survey (NHANES I) conducted from 1971 to 1975. The relation of the percentage of predicted DL(CO) to all-cause mortality was examined in a Cox proportional hazard model that included age, sex, race, current smoking status, systolic blood pressure, serum cholesterol, alcohol consumption, body mass index, percentage of predicted forced vital capacity (FVC), and the ratio of forced expiratory volume at 1 second (FEV1) to FVC. Mortality had a linear association with the percentage of predicted FVC (rate ratio (RR) = 1.12, 95% confidence interval (CI) 1.08-1.17, for a 10% decrement) and a

significantly nonlinear association with the percentage of predicted DL(CO) with an adverse effect that was clearly evident for levels below 85% of those predicted (RR = 1.24, 95% CI 1.12-1.37 for a 10% decrement). The relative hazard for the percentage of predicted DL(CO) below 85% was not modified by sex, smoking status, or exclusion of subjects with clinical respiratory disease on the initial examination. This association with the percentage of predicted DL(CO) was present among 3,005 subjects with FEV1 levels above 90% of those predicted. Thus, pulmonary diffusing capacity below 85% of predicted levels is a significant predictor of the all-cause mortality rate within the general US population independent of standard spirometry measures and even in the absence of apparent clinical respiratory disease.

Needham, LL; Hill, RH Jr; Ashley, DL; Pirkle, JL; Sampson, EJ (1995). The priority toxicant reference range study: interim report. *Env. Hlth. Persp.* 103 Suppl 3(Apr), 89-94. [adult; hazardous substances; middle age; NHANES-III; reference values].

Nordenberg, D; Yip, R; Binkin, NJ (1990). The effect of cigarette smoking on hemoglobin levels and anemia screening. *JAMA* 264(12, Sep 26), 1556-1559. [anemia, diagnosis; hemoglobins, analysis; NHANES II]

Paschal, DC (1995). Blood lead levels in the US population - Phase-1 of the third National Health and Nutrition Examination Survey. *JAMA* 274(2), 130. [blood lead levels; NHANES III; DHES].

Perez-Stable, EJ; Marin, BV; Marin, G; Brody, DJ; Benowitz, NL (1990). Apparent under reporting of cigarette consumption among Mexican American smokers [see comments]. *Am. J. Pub. Hlth.* 80(9, Sep), 1057-1061. [adult; aged; health surveys; HHANES; Hispanic Americans, psychology; self disclosure; smoking, psychology; DHES].

Perez-Stable, EJ; Marin, G; Marin, BV; Benowitz, NL (1992). Misclassification of smoking status by self-reported cigarette consumption. *Am. Rev. Resp. Dis.* 145(1, Jan), 53-57. [adult; aged; cotinine, blood; HHANES; self disclosure; smoking]

Perez-Stable, EJ; Benowitz, NL; Marin, G (1995). Is serum cotinine a better measure of cigarette smoking than self-report? *Prev. Med.* 24(2, Mar), 171-179. [adult; aged; body mass index; cotinine, blood; data collection, methods; HHANES; self disclosure; smoking, blood]

Perloff, BP; Rizek, RL; Haytowitz, DB; Reid, PR (1990). Dietary intake methodology. II. USDA's Nutrient Data Base for Nationwide Dietary Intake Surveys. *J. Nutr.* 120(S11)(Nov), 1530-1534. [agriculture; databases, factual; diet surveys; eating; NHANES II; NHANES III]

Perry, GS; Byers, T; Yip, R; Margen, S (1992). Iron nutrition does not account for the hemoglobin differences between blacks and whites. *J. Nutr.* 122(7, Jul), 1417-1424. [caucasoid race; hemoglobins, analysis; iron, blood; NHANES II].

Pirkle, JL; Brody, DJ; Gunter, EW; Kramer, RA; Paschal, DC; Flegal, KM; Matte, TD (1994):

The decline in blood lead levels in the United States. The National Health and Nutrition Examination Surveys (NHANES) [see comments]. *JAMA* 272(4, Jul 27), 284-291. [adolescence; adult; age factors; aged; child; child, preschool; cross-sectional studies; ethnic groups; health surveys; infant; lead, blood; middle age; NHANES-II; racial stocks; sex factors; DHES].

Pirkle, JL; Kaufmann, RB; Brody, DJ; Hickman, T; Gunter, EW; Paschal, DC (1998). Exposure of the U.S. population to lead, 1991-1994. *Environ Health Perspect* 106(11):745-50 (11, Nov), 745-750. [children; lead; NHANES III]
Blood lead measurements were obtained on 13,642 persons aged 1 year and older who participated in Phase 2 of the Third National Health and Nutrition Examination Survey (NHANES III) from 1991 through 1994. NHANES III is a national representative survey of the civilian, noninstitutionalized U.S. population. The overall mean blood lead level for the U.S. population aged 1 year and older was 2.3 microgram/dl, with 2.2% of the population having levels >=10 microgram/dl, the level of health concern for children. Among U.S. children aged 1-5 years, the mean blood lead level was 2.7 microgram/dl, and 890,000 of these children (4.4%) had elevated blood lead levels. Sociodemographic factors associated with higher blood lead levels in children were non-Hispanic black race/ethnicity, low income, and residence in older housing. The prevalence of elevated blood lead levels was 21.9% among non-Hispanic black children living in homes built before 1946 and 16.4% among children in low-income families who lived in homes built before 1946. Blood lead levels continue to decline in the U.S. population, but 890,000 children still have elevated levels. Public health efforts have been successful in removing lead from population-wide sources such as gasoline and lead-soldered food and drink cans, but new efforts must address the difficult problem of leaded paint, especially in older houses, as well as lead in dust and soil. Lead poisoning prevention programs should target high-risk persons, such as children who live in old homes, children of minority groups, and children living in families with low income.

Pletsch, PK (1991). Prevalence of cigarette smoking in Hispanic women of childbearing age. *Nurs. Res.* 40(2, Mar-Apr), 103-106. [adolescence; adult; age factors; HHANES; Hispanic Americans; smoking, epidemiology; smoking, ethnology]

Pletsch, PK (1994). Environmental tobacco smoke exposure among Hispanic women of reproductive age. *Pub. Hlth. Nurs.*11(4, Aug), 229-235. [adolescence; adult; age factors; child; environmental exposure; HHANES; Hispanic Americans; population surveillance; tobacco smoke pollution, statistical and numerical data; women's health].

Pocock, SJ; Shaper, AG; Ashby, D; Delves, HT; Clayton, BE (1988). The relationship between blood lead, blood pressure, stroke, and heart attacks in middle-aged British men. *Env. Hlth. Persp.* 78(Jun), 23-30. [adult; blood pressure, drug effects; cerebrovascular disorders, epidemiology; cerebrovascular disorders, etiology; Great Britain; health surveys; lead, blood; myocardial infarction, epidemiology; NHANES II]

Posner, BM; Cupples, LA; Franz, MM; Gagnon, DR (1993). Diet and heart disease risk factors in adult American men and women: The Framingham Offspring-Spouse nutrition studies. *Int. J. Epid.* 22(6), 1014-1025. [adult; aged; blood pressure; carbohydrate; carbohydrate intake; cardiovascular disease, epidemiology; cholesterol; cholesterol blood level; diet; dyslipidemia, epidemiology; eating habit; fat; fat intake; female; food intake; heart disease, epidemiology; human; hypertension, epidemiology; hypertension, rehabilitation; male; NHANES-II; obesity, epidemiology; risk factor; saturated fatty acid; sodium; sodium intake; United States; weight reduction]

Preston, AM (1991). Cigarette smoking-nutritional implications. *Progress in food and nutrition science.* 15(4), 183-217. [disease, etiology; minerals; NHANES-II; nutritional status; pregnancy; smoking, adverse effects; vitamins].

Roche, AF; Guo, S; Baumgartner, RN; Chumlea, WC; Ryan, AS; Kuczmarski, RJ (1990). Reference data for weight, stature, and weight/stature in Mexican Americans from the Hispanic Health and Nutrition Examination Survey (HHANES 1982-1984). *Clin. Nutr.* 51(5, Suppl, May), 917S-924S.(Includes 22 references.) [NHANES II; nutrition surveys; health; body weight; height; height-weight tables; children; adolescents; Mexican-Americans; DHES]

Romero-Gwynn, E; Gwynn, D (1991). Differential patterns of food-consumption among Mexican born and Mexican-Americans in the California HHANES sample. *FASEB J.* 5(6), 1665. [HHANES]

Russell, LB; Carson, JL; Taylor, WC; Milan,, E; Dey A; Jagannathan R (1998). Modeling all-cause mortality: projections of the impact of smoking cessation based on the NHEFS. NHANES I Epidemiologic Follow-up Study. *Am J Public Health* 88 (4, Apr), 630-636. [mortality; NHANES-I; NHEFS; smoking]
OBJECTIVES: A model that relates clinical risk factors to subsequent mortality was used to simulate the impact of smoking cessation. METHODS: Survivor functions derived from multivariate hazard regressions fitted to data from the first National Health and Nutrition Examination Survey (NHANES I) Epidemiologic Followup Study, a longitudinal survey of a representative sample of US adults, were used to project deaths from all causes. RESULTS: Validation tests showed that the hazard regressions agreed with the risk relationships reported by others, that projected deaths for baseline risk factors closely matched observed mortality, and that the projections attributed deaths to the appropriate levels of important risk factors. Projections of the impact of smoking cessation showed that the number of cumulative deaths would be 15% lower after 5 years and 11% lower after 20 years. CONCLUSIONS: The model produced realistic projections of the effects of risk factor modification on subsequent mortality in adults, Comparison of the projections for smoking cessation with estimates of the risk attributable to smoking published by the Centers for Disease Control and Prevention suggests that cessation could capture most of the benefit possible from eliminating smoking.

Sandler, RS; Lyles, CM; McAuliffe, C; Woosley, JT; Kupper LL (1993). Cigarette-smoking, alcohol, and the risk of colorectal adenomas. *Gastroenterology* 104(5), 1445-1451. [NHANES II]

Sandler, RS; Lyles, CM; Peipins, LA; McAuliffe, CA; Woosley, JT; Kupper, LL (1993). Diet and risk of colorectal adenomas - macronutrients, cholesterol, and fiber. *J. Natl. Cancer Inst.* 85 (11), 884-891. [adenoma; cholesterol; diet; fiber; NHANES].

Schlussel, YR; Schnall, PL; Zimbler, M; Warren, K; Pickering, TG (1990). The effect of work environments on blood pressure: evidence from seven New York organizations. *J. Hypertens.* 8(7, Jul), 679-685. [adult; blood pressure, physiology; cross-sectional studies; hypertension, epidemiology; middle age; NHANES-II; occupational diseases, epidemiology; occupations; work]

Schocken, DD; Arrieta, MI; Leaverton, PE; Ross, EA (1992). Prevalence and mortality rate of congestive heart failure in the United States. *J. Am. Coll. Cardiol.* 20(2, Aug), 301-306. [adult; age factors; heart failure, congestive, epidemiology; NHANES I].

Schwartz, J (1988). The relationship between blood lead and blood pressure in the NHANES II survey. *Env. Hlth. Persp.* 78(Jun), 15-22. [adult; aged; blood pressure, drug effects; lead, blood; NHANES II]

Schwartz, JD; Katz, SA; Fegley, RW; Tockman, MS (1988). Analysis of spirometric data from a national sample of healthy 6- to 24-year-olds (NHANES II). *Am. Rev. Respir. Dis.* 138(6, Dec), 1405-1414. [adolescence; adult; lung, physiology; NHANES-II; spirometry]

Schwartz, J; Katz, SA; Fegley, RW; Tockman, MS (1988). Sex and race differences in the development of lung function [see comments]. *Am. Rev. Respir. Dis.* 138(6, Dec), 1415-1421. [adolescence; adult; child; forced expiratory volume; forecasting; lung, physiology; NHANES-II; racial stocks; sex characteristics]

Schwartz, J (1989). Lung function and chronic exposure to air pollution: a cross-sectional analysis of NHANES II. *Env. Res.* 50(2, Dec), 309-321. [adolescence; adult; aged; air pollutants, adverse effects; air pollution, adverse effects; child; child, preschool; lung diseases, epidemiology; lung, physiology; NHANES II].

Schwartz ,J; Weiss, ST (1990). Dietary factors and their relation to respiratory symptoms. The second National Health and Nutrition Examination Survey. *Am. J. Epid.* 132(1, Jul), 67-76. [bronchial spasm, etiology; bronchitis, etiology; NHANES II].

Schwartz, J (1991). Lead, blood pressure, and cardiovascular disease in men and women. *Env. Hlth Pers.* 91(Feb), 71-75. [adult; aged; environmental pollutants, poisoning; heart enlargement, chemically induced; hypertension, chemically induced; lead poisoning, complications; NHANES II]

Schwartz, J; Otto, D (1991). Lead and minor hearing impairment. *Arch. Env. Hlth.* 46(5, Sep-Oct), 300-305. [hearing disorders, blood; Hispanic Americans; NHANES II]

Schwartz, J; Weiss, ST (1991). Host and environmental factors influencing the peripheral blood leukocyte count. *Am. J. Epid.* 134(12, Dec 15), 1402-1409. [leukocyte count; leukocytosis, epidemiology; NHANES II]

Schwartz, J; Weiss, ST (1992). Caffeine intake and asthma symptoms. *Ann. Epid.* 2(5), 627-635. [adult; asthma, epidemiology; coffee; human; methylxanthine; NHANES-II; normal human; tea; United States; wheezing]

Schwartz, J (1993). Particulate air pollution and chronic respiratory disease. *Env. Res.* 62(1, Jul), 7-13. [adolescence; adult; aged; air pollutants, toxicity; child; NHANES-I; respiratory tract diseases, chemically induced]

Schwartz, J; Weiss, ST (1993). Peripheral blood leukocyte count and respiratory symptoms. *Ann. Epid.* 3(1, Jan), 57-63. [bronchitis, blood; cough, blood; leukocytes; NHANES II]

Schwartz, J; Weiss, ST (1993). Prediction of respiratory symptoms by peripheral blood neutrophils and eosinophils in the First National Nutrition Examination Survey (NHANES I). *Chest* 104(4, Oct), 1210-1215. [adult; aged; cross-sectional studies; eosinophils; leukocyte count; neutrophils; NHANES-I; respiratory tract diseases, epidemiology].

Schwartz, J; Weiss, ST (1994). Cigarette smoking and peripheral blood leukocyte differentials. *Ann. Epidemiol.* 4(3, May), 236-242. [adult; aged; eosinophils, immunology; leukocyte count; NHANES-II; smoking cessation; smoking, immunology]

Schwartz, J; Weiss, ST (1994). Relationship between dietary vitamin C intake and pulmonary function in the first National Health and Nutrition Examination Survey (NHANES I). *Am. J. Clin. Nutr.* 59(1, Jan), 110-114. [adult; aged; ascorbic acid, administration and dosage; health surveys; lung, drug effects; lung, physiology; NHANES I]

Schwartz, J; Weiss, ST (1994). The relationship of dietary fish intake to level of pulmonary function in the first National Health and Nutrition Survey (NHANES I). *Eur. Respir. J.* 7(10, Oct), 1821-1824. [adult; aged; diet; fishes; forced expiratory volume; health surveys; middle age; NHANES-I, regression analysis; spirometry; United States]

Schwartz, J; Weiss, ST (1995). Relationship of skin test reactivity to decrements in pulmonary function in children with asthma or frequent wheezing. *Am. J. Respir. Crit. Care. Med.* 152(6 Pt 1, Dec), 2176-2180. [allergens; asthma, physiopathology; NHANES-II; respiratory mechanics; respiratory sounds, physiopathology; skin tests].

Shahar, E; Folsom, AR; Melnick, SL; Tockman, MS; Comstock, GW; Shimakawa, T; Higgins, MW; Sorlie, PD; Szklo, M (1994). Does dietary vitamin A protect against airway obstruction? The Atherosclerosis Risk in Communities (ARIC) Study Investigators. *Am. J. Respir. Crit. Care. Med.* 150(4, Oct), 978-982. [airway obstruction, epidemiology; airway obstruction, prevention and control; atherosclerosis, epidemiology; NHANES-I; Vitamin A, administration and dosage]

Shoff, SM; Newcomb, PA (1998): Diabetes, body size, and risk of endometrial cancer. *Am. J. Epid.* 148 (3, 1 Aug), 234-240. [cancer; diabetes; NHANES II]

Data from a population-based case-control study of Wisconsin women were used to evaluate the relation of diabetes to the risk of endometrial cancer on the basis of body mass index (BMI). Cases (n=723) were identified from a statewide tumor registry; controls (n=2,291) were selected randomly from population lists. Diabetes status, weight, height, and other factors were ascertained by telephone interview. Subjects were categorized as not overweight (BMI, <29.1), overweight (BMI, 29.1-31.9), or obese (BMI, >31.9) according to the BMI distribution of middle-aged white women in the second National Health and Nutrition Examination Survey. Joint associations between diabetes status, BMI, and endometrial cancer were evaluated using unconditional logistic regression models that controlled for age, parity, use of hormone replacement therapy, education, and smoking. Compared with persons without diabetes, those with diabetes had an adjusted odds ratio of 1.86 (95% confidence interval (CI) 1.37-2.52) for endometrial cancer. This association was modified by BMI (p interaction=0.04). Compared with non-overweight non-diabetic subjects, non-overweight and overweight women who reported diabetes had nonsignificant elevated risks of endometrial cancer (non-overweight, odds ratio (OR)=1.10, CI 0.66-1.86; overweight, OR=1.58, CI 0.81-3.05). In contrast, elevated risk estimates were observed for obese diabetic women (OR=2.95, CI 1.60-5.46). These data contradict earlier reports and suggest that diabetes confers no additional risk of endometrial cancer in women who are neither overweight nor obese.

Silbergeld, EK; Schwartz, J; Mahaffey, K (1988). Lead and osteoporosis: mobilization of lead from bone in postmenopausal women. *Env. Res.* 47(1, Oct), 79-94. [bone and bones, metabolism; lead, metabolism; NHANES II].

Smith, SA; Campbell, DR; Elmer, PJ; Martini, MC; Slavin, JL; Potter, JD (1995). The University of Minnesota Cancer Prevention Research Unit vegetable and fruit classification scheme (United States). *Cancer Causes & Control* 6(4), 292-302. [american diet; biological markers; beta-carotene; carcinogenesis; constituents; consumption; diet; epidemiologic methods; fruit; indoles; inhibition; juices; NHANES-II survey; metabolism; neoplasms; nutrition assessment; United States; vegetables].

Sorel, JE; Heiss, G; Tyroler, HA; Davis, WB; Wing, SB; Ragland, DR (1991). Black-white differences in blood pressure among participants in NHANES II: the contribution of blood lead. *Epid.* 2(5, Sep), 348-352. [blood pressure, physiology; caucasoid race; NHANES II].

Steenland, K; Sieber, K; Etzel, RA; Pechacek, T; Maurer, K (1998). Exposure to environmental tobacco smoke and risk factors for heart disease among never smokers in the third National Health and Nutrition Examination Survey. *Am J Epid.* 147 (10, 15 May), 932-939. [CHD; NHANES; smoking]

The relative risk of coronary artery disease among never smokers exposed to environmental tobacco smoke (ETS) versus never smokers not exposed to ETS is approximately 1.2 based on more than a dozen epidemiologic studies. Most of these studies have controlled for the major heart disease risk factors, but residual or uncontrolled confounding remains a possible explanation for the epidemiologic findings. The authors studied 3,338 never-smoking adults aged 17 years or older, who are representative of all US never smokers, in the 1988-1991 third National Health and Nutrition Examination Survey (NHANES III) to determine whether selected risk factors for heart disease differ between ETS-exposed and nonexposed persons. Both self-reported ETS exposure (at home and at work) and serum cotinine levels were available, the latter reflecting recent ETS exposure. After adjustments were made for age, sex, race, and education among adults aged 17 years or older, no significant differences were found between the ETS exposed and the nonexposed for any of 13 cardiovascular risk factors with the exception of dietary carotene, which was lower among the exposed. On the other hand, significant positive linear trends were found between serum cotinine and two risk factors (body mass index and alcohol consumption), and significant inverse trends were found with dietary carotene. There were also few differences between exposed and nonexposed never smokers among adults aged 40 years or older, who are most at risk of heart disease. In this group, however, there was an inverse linear trend between serum cotinine and high density lipoprotein cholesterol (p < 0.001). This finding could result from ETS exposure rather than be an indication of confounding; a similar inverse trend was found for children, confirming other results in the literature. Overall, these data suggest little potential for confounding by the heart disease risk factors studied here when ETS exposure is determined by self-report.

Stehr-Green, PA; Wohlleb, JC; Royce, W; Head, SL (1988). An evaluation of serum pesticide residue levels and liver function in persons exposed to dairy products contaminated with heptachlor. *JAMA* 259(3, Jan 15), 374-377. [adolescence; adult; aged; child; dairy products; food contamination; heptachlor, adverse effects; heptachlor, analysis; liver, drug effects; NHANES-II; pesticide residues, analysis].

Stehr-Green, PA (1989). Demographic and seasonal influences on human serum pesticide residue levels. J. Toxicol. *Env. Hlth.* 27(4), 405-421. [adolescence; adult; demography; NHANES-II; pesticide residues, analysis]

Stevens, RG; Jones, DY; Micozzi, MS; Taylor, PR (1988). Body iron stores and the risk of cancer [see comments]. *N. Engl. J. Med.* 319(16, Oct 20), 1047-1052. [ferritin, blood; follow-up studies; iron, metabolism; neoplasms, etiology; neoplasms, metabolism; NHANES-I; nutrition; risk-factors; serum albumin, analysis; sex factors].

Stevens, RG (1990). Iron and the risk of cancer. *Med. Oncol. Tumor Pharmacother.* 7(2-3), 177-181. [iron, adverse effects; liver neoplasms, epidemiology; NHANES I].

Subar, AF; Block, G; James, LD (1989). Folate intake and food sources in the US population. *Clin. Nutr.* 50(3, Sep), 508-516. [adult; aged; folic acid; middle age; NHANES-II; nutrition; nutrition surveys; United States]

Subar, AF; Harlan, LC; Mattson, ME (1990). Food and nutrient intake differences between smokers and non-smokers in the United States. *Am. J. Pub. Hlth.* 80(11, Nov), 1323-1329.

[adult; age factors; aged; blacks; caloric intake; diet; NHANES-II; smoking]

Swanson, CA; Jones, DY; Schatzkin, A; Brinton, LA; Ziegler, RG (1988). Breast cancer risk assessed by anthropometry in the NHANES I Epidemiological Follow-up Study. *Cancer Res.* 48(18, Sep 15), 5363-5367. [adult; aged; anthropometry; breast neoplasms, epidemiology; NHANES I; NHEFS]

Symanski, E; Hertz-Picciotto, I (1995). Blood lead levels in relation to menopause, smoking, and pregnancy history. *Am. J. Epid.* 141(11, Jun 1), 1047-1058. [adult; age factors; alcohol drinking, blood; lead, blood; menopause, blood; Mexican-Americans; NHANES-I; pregnancy, blood; reproductive history; smoking, blood].

Trout, D; Decker, J; Mueller, C; Bernert, JT; Pirkle, J (1998). Exposure of casino employees to environmental tobacco smoke. *J. Occup. Env. Med.* 40 (3, Mar), 270-276. [NHANES III; smoking]
Environmental and medical evaluations were performed to evaluate occupational exposure to environmental tobacco smoke (ETS) among casino employees. Air concentrations of both nicotine and respirable dust were similar to those published in the literature for other non-industrial indoor environments. The geometric mean serum cotinine level of the 27 participants who provided serum samples was 1.34 nanograms per milliliter (ng/mL) (pre-shift) and 1.85 ng/mL (post-shift). Both measurements greatly exceeded the geometric mean value of 0.65 ng/mL for participants in the Third National Health and Nutrition Examination Survey (NHANES III) who reported exposure to ETS at work. This evaluation demonstrates that a sample of employees working in a casino gaming area were exposed to ETS at levels greater than those observed in a representative sample of the US population, and that the serum and urine cotinine of these employees increased during the work shift.

Turkeltaub, PC; Gergen, PJ (1988). The prevalence of allergic and non-allergic respiratory symptoms in the United States population- data from the second National Health and Nutrition Examination Survey, 1976-80 (NHANES-II). *J. Allergy Clin. Immunol.* 81(1), 305. [NHANES II; DHES]

Turkeltaub, PC; Gergen, PJ (1991). Prevalence of upper and lower respiratory conditions in the US population by social and environmental factors: data from the second National Health and Nutrition Examination Survey, 1976 to 1980 (NHANES II). *Ann.Allergy* 67(2 Pt 1, Aug), 147-154. [age factors; NHANES-II; respiratory tract diseases, epidemiology; DHES].

Wagstaff, DJ (1993). Assessment of human exposure to toxic substances in food. *Tox. Subst. J.* 4(3), 184-198. [dietary intake; NHANES I]

Wallace, LA (1997). Human exposure and body burden for chloroform and other trihalomethanes. *Crit. Rev. in Env. Sci. and Tech.* 27, 113-194. [chloroform; NHANES; trihalomethanes]
Existing information on human exposure to chloroform and other trihalomethanes (THMs) in air,

water, and food is summarized. Three major surveys have collected data on chloroform levels in finished water at treatment plants. EPA's TEAM Studies have measured concentrations of THMs in residential drinking water and in personal, indoor, outdoor, and expired air from about 800 participants in eight cities. The Food and Drug Administration has surveyed chloroform levels in food and beverages. Recently, the Centers for Disease Control (CDC) have completed measuring blood levels of THMs in about 1000 participants in the National Health and Nutrition Examination Survey (NHANES). Exposure occurs through ingestion (drinking tap water and soft drinks and eating certain dairy foods), inhalation (breathing peak amounts of chloroform emitted during showers or baths, and lower levels in indoor air from other indoor sources), and dermal absorption (during showers, baths, and swimming). Each of these routes of exposure appear to be potentially substantial contributors to total exposure. The major source of exposure to chloroform is chlorination of water supplies. This results in exposure through ingestion of drinking water, but also through inhalation and skin absorption as a result of the myriad other uses of chlorinated water in the home: showers, baths, washing clothes and dishes, etc. Because chlorinated water supplies are used by bottling plants of soft drink manufacturers, even the chloroform found in beverages may be partially due to the chlorination of water supplies. Other sources of exposure, which can be important for specific groups of people, include chlorination of swimming pools, industrial production and use, and use of bleach during clothes washing. Wax, Y (1992). Collinearity diagnosis for a relative risk regression analysis: an application to assessment of diet-cancer relationship in epidemiological studies. *Stat. Med.* 11(10, Jul), 1273-1287. [breast neoplasms, etiology; diet; NHANES-I; NHEFS; regression analysis]

Whittemore, AS; DiCiccio, Y; Provenzano, G (1991). Urinary cadmium and blood pressure: results from the NHANES II survey. *Env. Hlth Persp.* 91(Feb), 133-140. [cadmium, urine; environmental pollutants, urine; NHANES II]

Whittemore, AS; Perlin, SA; DiCiccio, Y (1995). Chronic obstructive pulmonary disease in lifelong nonsmokers: results from NHANES. *Am. J. Pub. Hlth.* 85(5, May), 702-706. [aged; lung diseases, obstructive, epidemiology; NHANES I; NHANES II; NHANES III; smoking].

Wolff, CB; Portis, M; Wolff, H (1993). Birth weight and smoking practices during pregnancy among Mexican-American women. *Hlth. Care Women Int.* 14(3, May-Jun), 271-279. [birth weight; HHANES; Mexican-Americans; pregnancy, ethnology]

Wood, PR; Hidalgo, HA; Prihoda, TJ; Kromer, ME (1993). Hispanic children with asthma - morbidity. *Pediatrics* 91(1), 62-69. [HHANES].

Yong, LC; Brown, CC; Schatzkin, A; Dresser, CM; Slesinski, MJ; Cox, CS; Taylor, PR (1997). Intake of vitamins E, C, and A and risk of lung cancer - The NHANES I Epidemiologic Followup Study. *Am. J. Epid.* 146, 231-243. [lung cancer; NHANES I; NHEFS; vitamins] The relation between the dietary intake of vitamins E, C, and A (estimated by a 24-hour recall) and lung cancer incidence was examined in the first National Health and Nutrition Examination Survey Epidemiologic Followup Study cohort of 3,968 men and 6,100 women, aged 25-74 years. During a median follow-up period of 19 years (from 1971-1975 to 1992), 248 persons developed lung cancer. Adjusted for potential confounders using Cox proportional hazards regression methods with age as the underlying time variable, the relative risk of lung cancer for subjects in the highest quartile of vitamin C intake compared with those in the lowest quartile was 0.66 (95% confidence interval (CI) 0.45-0.96). For vitamin A intake, a protective effect was observed only for its fruit and vegetable component (carotenoids) among current smokers (relative risk = 0.49, 95% CI 0.29-0.84), but this was modified by the intensity of smoking (a statistically significant effect (relative risk = 0.33, 95% CI 0.13-0.84) was observed only for those in the lowest tertile of pack-years of smoking). The vitamin E intake-lung cancer relation was modified by the intensity of smoking with a significant protective effect confined to current smokers in the lowest tertile of pack-years of smoking (relative risk = 0.36, 95% CI 0.16-0.83). Overall, there was no additional protective effect of supplements of vitamins E, C, and A beyond that provided through dietary intake. When vitamin E, vitamin C, and carotenoid intakes were examined in combination, a strong protective effect was observed for those in the highest compared with those in the lowest quartile of all three intakes (relative risk = 0.32, 95% CI 0.14-0.74). These data provide support for a protective role of dietary vitamins E and C and of carotenoids against lung cancer risk but with a modification in effects by the intensity of cigarette exposure. While smoking avoidance is the most important behavior to reduce lung cancer risk, the daily consumption of a variety of fruits and vegetables that provides a combination of these nutrients and other potential protective factors may offer the best dietary protection against lung cancer.

Ziegler, RG; Ursin, G; Craft, NE; Subar, AF; Graubard, BI; Patterson, BH (1993). Does beta-carotene explain why reduced cancer risk is associated with vegetable and fruit intake? *Pennington Cen. Nutr. Ser.* 3, 352-371.(Literature review.) [beta-carotene; blood; carcinoma; carotenoids; chromatography; diet; disease prevention; food groups; food intake; fruit; literature reviews; NHANES-I; nutrient intake; nutrition research; risk; vegetables]

APPENDIX IX

Summaries of Recent EPA Studies Using NHANES Data

Title:	Use of NHANES Blood and Urine Biochemical Data in Evaluating Exposure for Risk Assessments and Response Actions at Superfund Sites

EPA Contact Person

Name: Elmer Akin

Phone Number: 404-562-8634

Office Affiliation: Office of Technical Services, Waste Management Div. (WMD), USEPA Region 4, Atlanta, GA

Description of Study

1) Which NHANES did you use? ☐ **NHANES-I**   ☐ **NHANES-II** ☐ **NHANES-III** ☐ **HHANES**
 ▶ **NHANES99+** (*check to the left of each appropriate box*)

2) Characteristics of the study group (*e.g., age, gender, race/ethnicity, region of country*)**:**
All the NHANES99+ subjects, plus any breakouts of the population data that can be developed just for the southeastern part of the U.S.. Subjects are classified by age, race, gender, etc.

3) Detailed description of the goals/purpose and approach of the study:
Blood and urine levels of environmental chemicals (e.g., pesticides, organochlorines, metals) in U.S. random population samples from NHANES are used as screening levels for comparison with data from local populations exposed to hazardous waste sites (Superfund sites). Blood and urine levels of these chemicals in local populations are compared to the mean levels derived from NHANES99+. In the future, as data permit, this analysis will be refined by stratifying both the local populations and the NHANES subjects by age, race, sex, etc. and then comparing the blood and urine levels by these categories.

4) What statistical methods and models are you using? Include a brief summary of how you present the results. If appropriate, attach sample tables and/or charts.
We calculate mean values and distribution statistics by age, race, gender, etc. for the blood and urine levels of the environmental chemicals evaluated in NHANES99+.

5) If you use NHANES data without publishing documents, include a brief description of these cases.   (e.g., use of raw NHANES data and/or results from published NHANES studies to support setting pesticide tolerances on food, or to support setting air quality standards for ambient pollutants.):
The NHANES values are used as an input parameter in determining potential risk to local populations around hazardous waste sites and Superfund sites and in determining the need for regulatory action. In the future, these comparisons of environmental chemicals in blood and urine of local population and NHANES subjects will be used to determine the urgency and priority of response actions.

Citation and Abstract/Executive Summary

Citation:

Dates for Completed Studies:

Starting Date: **Ending Date:**

Information for Work in Progress:

Anticipated Product(s):
Tentative Completion Date(s):

Title:	NHANES-III/HHANES Pesticide Epidemiology Study

EPA Contact Person

Name: Ruth Allen   **Office Affiliation:** Office of Pesticide Programs (OPP), Health Effects Div (HED), Office of Prevention, Pesticides and Toxic Substances (OPPTS), Washington, DC

Phone Number: 703-305-7191

Description of Study

1) Which NHANES did you use? ☐ NHANES-I   ☐ NHANES-II X ☐ NHANES-III X ☐ HHANES
▶ NHANES99+ *(check to the left of each appropriate box)*

2) Characteristics of the study group *(e.g., age, gender, race/ethnicity, region of country)*:
NHANES subjects are classified by the following variables: socio-demographic (e.g., age, education, gender, race/ethnicity, poverty-income ratio, place of residence), personal life style (e.g., tobacco & alcohol use, # rooms in home, # people in home, year house was built), medical/reproduction (e.g., general health status, access to health care, blood group parameters), environmental (e.g., source of drinking water), occupational (e.g., usual & current occupation & business or industry), diet (e.g., foods eaten), and regional variation (e.g., state, county, census region, urban/urban fringe or rural residence). Analysis of pesticides groups focused only on adults 20-59 years old, & included 978 subjects from NHANES-III & 2008 Mexican-Americans from HHANES who had urinary pesticide measurements.

3) Detailed description of the goals/purpose and approach of the study: Determine prevalence of pesticide exposure biomarkers among subgroups of NHANES-III and HHANES, as noted above, & determine if there are statistically significant risks of exposure associated with these subgroup characteristics. OPP uses NHANES data to: a) validate aggregate and cumulative risk models; b) characterize exposures to single & multiple pesticide parent compounds, or their metabolites, in various human subgroups at various points in time; c) improve understanding of how exposure to pesticide metabolites affects human health; d) examine probable routes of pesticide exposures, including through residues in food, drinking water & in occupational & residential settings, for both aggregate and cumulative exposures. These analyses will provide OPP with valid & reliable information on environmental exposures and body burdens for the set of pesticides assessed in NHANES-III, HHANES, and NHANES 99+ so that risk managers and assessors can make decisions based on actual human data.

4) What statistical methods and models are you using? Include a brief summary of how you present the results. If appropriate, attach sample tables and/or charts.
Simple frequency tables, univariate analysis, odds ratio, t-tests and maximum likelihood methods.

5) If you use NHANES data without publishing documents, include a brief description of these cases. (e.g., use of raw NHANES data and/or results from published NHANES studies to support setting pesticide tolerances on food, or to support setting air quality standards for ambient pollutants.):
Based on urinary pesticide levels in NHANES-III, HHANES, and eventually NHANES 99+ subjects, OPP will estimate the underlying distribution of possible pesticide exposures in the U.S. population. This underlying distribution will be compared to EPA's oral Reference Dose (RfD) values for specific pesticides to evaluate the adequacy of protection under current regulations. In instances where pesticide metabolites are elevated above the minium detectable level, OPP will use the NHANES subpopulation characteristics to help identify segments of the U.S. population potentially at high risk of exposure to these pesticides.

Results support OPP on-going efforts to use more real human data in models for aggregate and cumulative risk assessments. Conclusions drawn from NHANES-III, HHANES, and eventually NHANES99+ pesticide data can be used to cross-check and validate results from other NHANES surveys (i.e., NHANES 03+) and from published biomonitoring data from other large population-based environmental epidemiology and environmental health studies.

Citation and Abstract/Executive Summary:

Citation:
1) Mage, D., Allen, R., Gondy, G., Smith, W., Barr, D., Needham, L., (2001). Estimating Pesticide Exposures of NHANES-III participants. Presentation given at International Society for Exposure Assessment (ISEA) Conference in South Carolina, 2001.
2) Allen, R., Werner, E., Gondy, G., Mage, D., (2000). The NHANES-III/ HHANES Pesticide Epidemiology (PEPI) Study: Examination of High End Exposure. Presentation given at American Public Health Association (APHA) Conference in Boston 2000.
3) Allen, R., Werner, E.,(1999). The NHANES III/HHANES Pesticide Epidemiology Study. Presentation given at American Public Health Association (APHA) Conference in Chicago 1999.

Dates for Completed Studies:

Starting Date: **Ending Date:**

Information for Work in Progress:

Anticipated Product(s): Reports on NHANES-III and HHANES chemical-specific statistics for organophosphates, carbamates, phenoxyacetic acids, organochlorines and fungicides. Reports on comparison of chemical groups and specific chemicals of interest in NHANES data, plus comparisons with data in the open literature, population-based analyses, unresolved statistical and methodological issues for population- based risk assessment and recommendations for future NHANES analyses.

Tentative Completion Date(s): Chemical specific reports for 2,-4 D, lindane and methyl parathion, completed in 2001. Reports for chlorpyrifos, propoxur, carbofuran, carbaryl planned for completion in 2002. In 2002 the NHANES analysis team will complete papers on maximum likelihood estimation methods and on reclassification of NHANES occupation codes.

Abstracts:
1) Mage, D., Allen, R., Gondy, G., Smith, W., Barr, D., Needham, L.., (2001). Estimating Pesticide Exposures of NHANES-III participants. Presentation given at International Society for Exposure Assessment (ISEA) Conference in South Carolina, 2001.

The Third National Health and Nutrition Examination Survey (NHANES-III) collected a single urine sample for pesticide analysis from almost 1000 subjects during the period 1988-1994. The subjects were male and female volunteers from a national probability sample, with ages 20 to 59. We assume that the choice to donate or not donate urine was independent of the subject's pesticide exposure variables, so that the urine samples are equivalent to a national probability sample. The urine was analyzed for 12 pesticide residues that correspond to more than 30 different possible parent compounds. These data, reported as mg residue/liter (mg/L) are only indicative of an exposure if the values are above the minimum detectable level (MDL) for each residue. Because volumetric urine production depends upon the variable quantity of fluids people ingest prior to the sample collection, it is necessary to normalize the urinary pesticide excretion rates by dividing by the urinary excretion rate of creatinine (gCr/L) to provide a value of mg /gCr.

Each individual excretes creatinine at their own constant daily rate, a function of their gender, age, height and weight, muscularity, and renal-related health status (gCr/day). From the subject questionnaire data we estimate the individual's daily creatinine excretion rate and multiplying it by mg/gCr we obtain an estimate of the daily excretion rate of the pesticide residue. Using stoichiometry and moiety data, we analyze and report the constant daily intake of the most likely parent pesticide of the residue that would lead to a constant daily urinary excretion rate of residue equal to the measured values. We divide by the subject's recorded body weight to obtain the equivalent dose rate in mg/kg/day for comparison to the reference dose (RfD) established by EPA for each pesticide.
We fit the distribution of estimated dose rates by a Johnson S_B (4-parameter lognormal) model. A major methodological difficulty in fitting these data is the large number of below MDL values (BMDL). Each BMDL (mg/L) corresponds to a value less than a variable amount of residue per gram creatinine. We fit the S_B model using the exact and MDL values by the method of maximum likelihood estimation (MLE) to predict the fraction of the population of the U.S. that is expected to be exposed to the pesticide at or above the RfD. People are exposed to pesticides in the air, water and diet by ingestion and dermal contact. However, when pesticides degrade in the environment from microbial activity or sunlight, these residues remain in the environment and can also be inhaled or ingested in water and food. Given these considerations, the model results show that less than 1 person in 1000 is expected to be exposed to the parent pesticide at or above the RfD. We recommend that the ongoing NHANES surveys continue to report, at least, the same 12 pesticide residues so that changes in estimated exposures over time can be obtained to evaluate the effect of regulation. We also recommend that a 24-hour total urine collection be instituted, to replace the estimates of daily creatinine and pesticide-residue excretion with measured values.

The overall significance of this approach is that we make use of the complete data set, including BMDL values, to estimate the underlying distribution of possible pesticide exposures in the U.S. We compare these exposures to the RfD to evaluate the adequacy of protection.

2) Allen, R., Werner, E., Gondy, G., Mage, D., (2000). The NHANES-III/ HHANES Pesticide Epidemiology (PEPI) Study: Examination of High End Exposure. Presentation given at American Public Health Association (APHA) Conference in Boston 2000.

The NHANES III/Hispanic HANES Pesticide Epidemiology (PEPI) Study is designed to analyze the prevalence of pesticide biomarkers among samples of the survey populations from the National Health and Nutrition Examination Survey III (NHANES) and the Hispanic Health and Nutrition Examination Survey (HHANES). The distribution percentiles of urinary metabolites of more than 20 pesticides have been determined. These distributions enabled us to identify subjects with high serum and urinary levels of pesticide analytes who are at potential risk for pesticide-related illnesses. This analysis focuses a detailed examination of individuals at the high end of exposure both at the 95th and 99th percentiles. Among the 1,018 people in the NHANES III pesticide sample, six had high values for more than one analyte: two females, one aged 40-49 who is a non-Hispanic white, and one aged 20-29 who is Mexican-American. The four males include two non-Hispanic blacks between 40-49 years of age and two non-Hispanic whites between 30-39 years. The results are useful for efforts underway to use more real data in support of models for aggregate and cumulative risk assessments. The conclusions also contribute to comparisons across NHANES surveys and with published biomonitoring data from other large population-based environmental epidemiology and environmental health studies.

3) Allen, R., Werner, E.,(1999). The NHANES III/HHANES Pesticide Epidemiology Study. Presentation given at American Public Health Association (APHA) Conference in Chicago 1999.

The NHANES-III/Hispanic HANES Pesticide Epidemiology (PEPI) Study is designed to analyze the prevalence of pesticide biomarkers among samples of the survey populations from the National Health and Nutrition Examination Survey III (NHANES) and the Hispanic Health and Nutrition Examination Survey (HHANES). The distribution percentiles of urinary metabolites of more than 20 pesticides will be determined for the NHANES III and HHANES sample populations, and will be analyzed in relation to the sample population' sociodemographic, geographic, occupational, and other personal characteristics. The pesticides examined include carbamates; phenoxyacetic acid herbicides; fungicides; and organochlorines. These compounds have been prioritized to meet EPA's regulatory obligations in the implementation of its Office of Pesticide Programs. Elevated detectable levels of metabolites associated with sample populations' characteristics will enable the EPA to identify segments of the U.S. population at high risk exposure to pesticides.

Title:	Estimates of body weight for water program exposure and risk assessment

EPA Contact Person

Name: Denis Borum and Helen Jacobs   **Office Affiliation:** Office of Science & Technology (OST), Office of Water (OW), Washington, DC

Phone Number: 202-260-8996 (Denis); 202-260-5412 (Helen)

Description of Study

1) Which NHANES did you use? ☐ NHANES-I   ☐ NHANES-II   ☑ NHANES-III   ☐ HHANES
    ☐ NHANES99+ (*check to the left of each appropriate box*)

2) Characteristics of the study group (*e.g., age, gender, race/ethnicity, region of country*)**:**
  Groups classified by age and gender

3) Detailed description of the goals/purpose and approach of the study:
OW revised its "Methodology for Deriving Ambient Water Quality Criteria for the Protection of Human Health" reflecting many scientific advances since its original publication in 1980. The NHANES analysis was conducted in order to provide body weight recommendations for various age and gender categories based on the most recent available data.

4) What statistical methods and models are you using? Include a brief summary of how you present the results. If appropriate, attach sample tables and/or charts.
Tabulations of national estimates of body weight in kilograms by age and gender are provided for selected age categories. The statistical sampling weights used in NHANES-III for the national estimates are the "examined sample final weights". These weights apply to all persons examined in the Mobile Examination Centers or at home.

5) If you use NHANES data without publishing documents, include a brief description of these cases.   (e.g., use of raw NHANES data and/or results from published NHANES studies to support setting pesticide tolerances on food, or to support setting air quality standards for ambient pollutants.):
Incorporated into guidance document and will be used to develop Water Quality Criteria.

Citation and Abstract/Executive Summary

Citation: USEPA. 2000. Methodology for Deriving Ambient Water Quality Criteria for the Protection of Human Health (2000). Office of Science and Technology, Office of Water. EPA-822-B-00-004. October

Dates For Completed Studies:

Starting Date: **Ending Date:** October 2002

Information for Work in Progress:

Anticipated Product(s): A Technical Support Document on Exposure Assessment to provide greater details on the Methodology, including finer age categories for body weight.

Tentative Completion Date(s): September 2002.

Title:	Analysis of Serological Responses to Cryptosporidium Antigen Among NHANES III Participants

EPA Contact Person

Name: Rebecca Calderon

Phone Number: 919-966-0617

Office Affiliation: Human Studies Division (HSD), National Health & Environmental Effects Research Laboratory (NHEERL), Research Triangle Park, NC

Description of Study

1) Which NHANES did you use? ☐ **NHANES-I** ☐ **NHANES-II** ☒ **NHANES-III** ☐ **HHANES**
☐ **NHANES99+** *(check to the left of each appropriate box)*

2) Characteristics of the study group *(e.g., age, gender, race/ethnicity, region of country)*:
Surplus sera from subjects within seven of the NHANES-III primary sampling units (PSUs) were used. These seven geographic areas were selected because they differed in their sources and treatment of drinking water. First, the PSUs were selected, then sera were selected randomly from subjects living in each PSU.

3) Detailed description of the goals/purpose and approach of the study: The objective of the study was to see if intensity of serum antibody response to Cryptosporidium was related to a PSU and therefore the primary source and treatment of drinking water. Each PSU was composed of one or more adjacent counties. The PSUs were chosen based on their source water characteristics.

4) What statistical methods and models are you using? Include a brief summary of how you present the results. If appropriate, attach sample tables and/or charts. Multivariate analysis of the observed intensity of serological response to the Cryptosporidium antigens was conducted using a Tobit model. Because of the multistage design of the NHANES survey, the analyses were stratified first by the PSU and then by family within the PSU. Data are presented in tabular form.

5) If you use NHANES data without publishing documents, include a brief description of these cases. (e.g., use of raw NHANES data and/or results from published NHANES studies to support setting pesticide tolerances on food, or to support setting air quality standards for ambient pollutants.):

Citation and Abstract/Executive Summary

Citation: Analysis of Serological Responses to *Cryptosporidium* Antigen Among NHANES III Participants

Dates for Completed Studies:

Starting Date: October 1993   **Ending Date:** January 31, 2002

Information for Work in Progress:

Anticipated Product(s): Journal article
Tentative Completion Date(s): Draft journal article being revised based on reviews for clearance.

Abstract

This study related the intensity of serological responses to two *Cryptosporidium* antigen groups with the city of residence, family, age, sex and other characteristics of study participants for 1356 NHANES III participants from seven of the Survey's primary sampling units (PSUs). The PSUs differed in their primary source and treatment of drinking water. The mean intensity of serological responses differed by PSU but not by family unit within the PSU. Increasing age, female sex, Black race, serological response to *Toxoplasma* and larger family size were associated with a more intense response to both antigen markers ($p<0.05$). Other race, residing in a major metropolitan area and seropositivity of Hispanics for hepatitis A were also associated with a more intense response to the 15/17-kDa marker ($p<0.05$). Results suggest that *Cryptosporidium* transmission occurs within households, especially in large families. No associations were detected between the intensity of serological response and health status.

Title:	Examination of Risk Factors for Respiratory Effects in Children: Use of Respiratory Health and EPA Air Monitoring Data. Part I: Effect of Asthma Status and Household Environmental Exposures on Lung Function of Children and Adolescents.

EPA Contact Person

Name: Robert Chapman   **Office Affiliation:** National Center for Environmental Assessment (NCEA), Office of Research & Development. Research Triangle Park, NC

Phone Number: 919-541-4492

Description of Study

1) Which NHANES did you use? ☐ NHANES-I   ☐ NHANES-II   ▶ NHANES-III   ☐ HHANES
☐ NHANES99+

2) Characteristics of the study group *(e.g., age, gender, race/ethnicity, region of country)*:
All 8-16 year-old subjects who had spirometric lung function testing.

3) Detailed description of the goals/purpose and approach of the study:
 1. Ascertain effects of active and inactive asthma, and of the household environmental factors passive smoking, cooking with a gas stove, and presence of a dog or cat, on children's and adolescents' lung function.
 2. Compare sensitivities of different lung function metrics (i.e., FEV1, FVC, MMEF) in detecting effects of asthma and household environmental factors.

4) What statistical methods and models are you using? Include a brief summary of how you present the results. If appropriate, attach sample tables and/or charts.
 Linear regression models using SUDAAN software. This gives the same effects estimates (betas) as does simple linear regression, but also employs generalized estimating equations to adjust standard errors and p-values for non-independence arising from clustering in the data.

5) If you use NHANES data without publishing documents, include a brief description of these cases. (e.g., use of raw NHANES data and/or results from published NHANES studies to support setting pesticide tolerances on food, or to support setting air quality standards for ambient pollutants.):

Citation and Abstract/Executive Summary

Citation:

For Completed Studies, Provide the Following Dates:

Starting Date: **Ending Date:**

Work in Progress, Provide the Following Information:

Anticipated Product(s): Peer-reviewed journal article.
Tentative Completion Date(s): June 2002.

Title:	Examination of Risk Factors for Respiratory Effects in Children: Use of Respiratory Health and EPA Air Monitoring Data. Part II: Effects of Ethnicity on Lung Function in Children and Adolescents

EPA Contact Person

Name: Robert Chapman   **Office** Affiliation: National Center for Environmental Assessment (NCEA), Office of Research & Development. Research Triangle Park, NC

Phone Number: 919-541-4492

Description of Study

1) Which NHANES did you use? ☐ NHANES-I   ☐ NHANES-II   ▶ NHANES-III   ☐ HHANES
    ☐ NHANES99+ (*please check to the left of each appropriate box*)

2) Characteristics of the study group (*e.g., age, gender, race/ethnicity, region of country*):
All 8-16 year-old subjects who had spirometric lung function testing.

3) Detailed description of the goals/purpose and approach of the study:
Ascertain effects of ethnicity on lung function in children and adolescents. Model-adjusted lung function will be compared among non-Hispanic whites, non-Hispanic blacks, and Mexican-Americans. Comparative assessment of Puerto-Rican Americans' lung function will also be conducted, to the extent that the NHANES III data allow.

4) What statistical methods and models are you using? Include a brief summary of how you present the results. If appropriate, attach sample tables and/or charts.
Linear regression models using SUDAAN software. This gives the same effects estimates (betas) as does simple linear regression, but also employs generalized estimating equations to adjust standard errors and p-values for non-independence arising from clustering in the data.

5) If you use NHANES data without publishing documents, include a brief description of these cases. (e.g., use of raw NHANES data and/or results from published NHANES studies to support setting pesticide tolerances on food, or to support setting air quality standards for ambient pollutants.):

Citation and Abstract/Executive Summary

Citation:

For Completed Studies, Provide the Following Dates:

Starting Date: **Ending Date:**

Work in Progress, Provide the Following Information:

Anticipated Product(s): Peer-reviewed journal article.
Tentative Completion Date(s): June 2002.

Title:	Examination of Risk Factors for Respiratory Effects in Children: Use of Respiratory Health and EPA Air Monitoring Data. Part III: Risk Factors for Asthma in Children and Adolescents

EPA Contact Person

Name: Robert Chapman **Office** Affiliation: National Center for Environmental Assessment (NCEA), Office of Research & Development. Research Triangle Park, NC

Phone Number: 919-541-4492

Description of Study

1) Which NHANES did you use? ☐ **NHANES-I**   ☐ **NHANES-II** ☑ **NHANES-III** ☐ **HHANES**
  ☐ **NHANES99+** (*please check to the left of each appropriate box*)

2) Characteristics of the study group (*e.g., age, gender, race/ethnicity, region of country*)**:**
All subjects ages 0-16 years.

3) Detailed description of the goals/purpose and approach of the study:
 Ascertain effects of host and environmental factors on prevalence of asthma in children and adolescents. Host factors of interest include age, gender, ethnicity, and atopic-allergic status. Environmental factors of interest include passive smoking, cooking with a gas stove, and presence of pets in the household.

4) What statistical methods and models are you using? Include a brief summary of how you present the results. If appropriate, attach sample tables and/or charts.
 Logistic regression models, adjusted for cluster effects with generalized estimating equations (SUDAAN software or SAS GENMOD procedure).

5) If you use NHANES data without publishing documents, include a brief description of these cases.   (e.g., use of raw NHANES data and/or results from published NHANES studies to support setting pesticide tolerances on food, or to support setting air quality standards for ambient pollutants.):

Citation and Abstract/Executive Summary

Citation:

For Completed Studies, Provide the Following Dates:

Starting Date: **Ending Date:**

Work in Progress, Provide the Following Information:

Anticipated Product(s): Peer-reviewed journal article.
Tentative Completion Date(s): April 2002.

Title:	Mercury (Hg)

EPA Contact Person

Name: Chuck French Emission

Office Affiliation: Office of Air Quality Planning and Standards (OAQPS), Standards Div. (ESD), Office of Air and Radiation (OAR), Research Triangle Park, NC

Phone Number: 919-541-0467

Description of Study

1) **Which NHANES did you use?** ☐ **NHANES-I** ☐ **NHANES-II** ☐ **NHANES-III** ☐ **HHANES** ▶ **NHANES99+** (*check to the left of each appropriate box*)

2) **Characteristics of the study group** (*e.g., age, gender, race/ethnicity, region of country*)**:** Women of childbearing age (16-49 years old) and young children (1-5 years old).

3) **Detailed description of the goals/purpose and approach of the study:** Blood and hair Hg levels from NHANES 1999 were used to help support a regulatory determination for Hg emissions from electric utilities as well as several other Hg projects (e.g., Mercury Action Plan, PBT Monitoring Strategy). These data have proven to be very useful and informative and support our technical and policy efforts with Hg.

4) **What statistical methods and models are you using? Include a brief summary of how you present the results. If appropriate, attach sample tables and/or charts.** Data and statistical results presented in the publication on March 2, 2001 in the CDC's Morbidity & Mortality Weekly Report (MMWR) (see below) are used in this work. The MMWR presents the data as geometric mean and percentiles (10th, 25th, 50th, 75th, 90th) for both the women and children for blood Hg and for hair Hg.

5) **If you use NHANES data without publishing documents, include a brief description of these cases. (e.g., use of raw NHANES data and/or results from published NHANES studies to support setting pesticide tolerances on food, or to support setting air quality standards for ambient pollutants.):** NHANES results (as reported in the MMWR article) were used with lots of other information to support the general conclusion that Hg in the environment and Hg exposures for the U.S. human population are of concern, and there is a need for emissions reductions. The amount of emissions reductions needed to decrease environmental exposures was not quantified, nor were estimate was made of Hg environmental exposure due to utility emissions. The NHANES results have been used in various briefings, posters, draft reports, etc.... to support various Hg efforts and to present information on Hg exposures.

Citation and Abstract/Executive Summary

Citation: Blood and Hair Mercury Levels in Young Children and Women of Childbearing Age --- United States, 1999. *MMWR, March 2, 2001,* Vol 50, No 08;140. (Contributing authors from EPA included Kate Mahaffey and Chuck French) http://www.cdc.gov/mmwr/preview/mmwrhtml/mm5008a2.htm

Dates for Completed Studies:

Starting Date: **Ending Date:**

Information for Work in Progress:

Anticipated Product(s): Various
Tentative Completion Date(s): Uncertain

Abstract:

Blood and Hair Mercury Levels in Young Children and Women of Childbearing Age --- United States, 1999.

Mercury (Hg), a heavy metal, is widespread and persistent in the environment. Exposure to hazardous Hg levels can cause permanent neurologic and kidney impairment (1--3). Elemental or inorganic Hg released into the air or water becomes methylated in the environment where it accumulates in animal tissues and increases in concentration through the food chain. The U.S. population primarily is exposed to methyl mercury by eating fish. Methyl mercury exposures to women of childbearing age are of great concern because a fetus is highly susceptible to adverse effects. This report presents preliminary estimates of blood and hair Hg levels from the 1999 National Health and Nutrition Examination Survey (NHANES 1999) and compares them with a recent toxicologic review by the National Research Council (NRC). The findings suggest that Hg levels in young children and women of childbearing age generally are below those considered hazardous. These preliminary estimates show that approximately 10% of women have Hg levels within one tenth of potentially hazardous levels indicating a narrow margin of safety for some women and supporting efforts to reduce methyl mercury exposure.

CDC's NHANES is a continuous survey of the health and nutritional status of the U.S. civilian, noninstitutionalized population with each year of data constituting a representative population sample. A household interview and a physical examination were conducted for each survey participant. During the physical examination, blood was collected by venipuncture for all persons aged >1 year and hair samples, consisting of approximately 100 strands, were cut from the occipital position of the head of children aged 1--5 years and women aged 16--49 years. Whole blood specimens were analyzed for total Hg and inorganic Hg for children aged 1--5 years and women aged 16--49 years by automated cold vapor atomic absorption spectrophotometry in CDC's trace elements laboratory. The detection limit was 0.2 parts per billion (ppb) for total Hg and 0.4 ppb for inorganic Hg (4). Hairs of 0.6 inches (1.5 cm) closest to the scalp (approximately 1 month's growth) were analyzed for total Hg concentration using cold vapor atomic fluorescence spectroscopy (5). The limit of detection for total Hg in hair varied by analytic batch; the maximum limit of detection (0.1 parts per million [ppm]) was used in these analyses. Blood Hg levels less than the limit of detection were assigned a value equal to the detection limit divided by the square root of two for calculation of geometric mean values. The geometric mean total blood Hg concentration for all women aged 16--49 years and children aged 1--5 years was 1.2 ppb and 0.3 ppb, respectively; the 90th percentile of blood Hg for women and children was 6.2 ppb and 1.4 ppb, respectively (Table 1). Almost all inorganic Hg levels were undetectable; therefore, these measures indicate blood methyl mercury levels. The 90th percentile of hair Hg for women and children was 1.4 ppm and 0.4 ppm, respectively. Geometric mean values were not calculated for hair Hg values.

Reported by: Center for Food Safety and Applied Nutrition, Food and Drug Administration. US Environmental Protection Agency. National Energy Technology Laboratory, Dept of Energy. National Marine Fisheries Laboratory, National Oceanic and Atmospheric Administration. National Center for Health Statistics; National Center for Environmental Health, CDC.

Title:	Methyl Ethyl Ketone (MEK) (also called 2-butanone)

EPA Contact Person

Name: Chuck French   **Office Affiliation:** Office of Air Quality Planning and Standards (OAQPS), Emission Standards Div. (ESD), Office of Air and Radiation (OAR), Research Triangle Park, NC
Phone Number: 919-541-0467

Description of Study

1) Which NHANES did you use? ☐ **NHANES-I** ☐ **NHANES-II** ▶ **NHANES-III** ☐ **HHANES**
   ☐ **NHANES99+** (*check to the left of each appropriate box*)

2) **Characteristics of the study group** (*e.g., age, gender, race/ethnicity, region of country*)**:**
Unstratified sample of adults 20-59 years of age. Variables such as age and race were not used in the analysis.

3) **Detailed description of the goals/purpose and approach of the study:** Blood MEK measurements from NHANES III were used to determine background levels in humans due to environmental exposures plus normal metabolism. These data were considered along with other information to help evaluate a petition submitted to EPA by the Chemical Industry to delist MEK from the Clean Air Act List of Hazardous Air Pollutants.

4) **What statistical methods and models are you using? Include a brief summary of how you present the results. If appropriate, attach sample tables and/or charts.** Raw NHANES-III data were not used. Instead, data and statistical results were taken from 2 publications (Ashley, et al., 1994 and Churchill, et al. 2001, see below for full citations). The results were as follows: n = 1101 adults; median MEK blood level = 5.4 ppb; mean = 7 ppb; 5th %ile = 2 ppb; 95th %ile = 17 ppb. A positive association was observed for alcohol, smoking, & exposure to moth balls & pressure-treated wood, but, these factors do not appear to account for average exposures.

5) **If you use NHANES data without publishing documents, include a brief description of these cases. (e.g., use of raw NHANES data and/or results from published NHANES studies to support setting pesticide tolerances on food, or to support setting air quality standards for ambient pollutants.):** Published MEK data were used in the evaluation of the delist petition. When a final decision on the petition has been made, it will be published in the Federal Register and will reference the NHANES data and studies. These NHANES results are one of several important factors in the overall review and analysis of the petition. Various calculations were made to compare the NHANES blood levels with those levels one might expect to see in a population from chronic exposure to MEK at the level of EPA's Inhalation Reference Concentration (RfC). The mean blood levels from NHANES were about 2 times higher than the levels expected from chronic exposure at the RfC. This was useful information for the analysis and raised questions about the RfC, natural levels of MEK, etc.

Citation and Abstract/Executive Summary

Citation:

For Completed Studies, Provide the Following Dates:

Starting Date: **Ending Date:**

Work in Progress, Provide the Following Information:

Anticipated Product(s): Federal Register Notice
Tentative Completion Date(s): Year 2002

References Used to Estimate MEK Background Levels for this Work:

1. Ashley, et al. 1994. Blood Concentrations of Volatile Organic Compounds in a Non-occupationally Exposed US Population and in Groups with Suspected Exposures. *Clin. Chem.* 40/7, 1401-1404 (1994).
2. Churchill, J.E., Kaye, W.E. 2001. Recent Exposures and Blood Volatile Organic Compound Levels in a Large Population-Based Sample. *Archives of Environmental Health.* March/April 2001. Vol. 56 (No. 2).

Title:	Environmental Risk Factors for Presence of *Cryptosporidium parvum* Antibodies in Human Serum

EPA Contact Person

Name: Elizabeth Hilborn   **Office Affiliation:** Epidemiology & Biomarkers Branch, Human Studies Division, National Health & Environmental Effects Research Laboratory (NHEERL), Research Triangle Park, NC

Phone Number: 919- 966-0658

Description of Study

1) **Which NHANES did you use?** ☐ **NHANES-I**   ☐ **NHANES-II**   ☒ **NHANES-III**   ☐ **HHANES**
    ☐ **NHANES99+** *(check to the left of each appropriate box)*

2) **Characteristics of the study group** *(e.g., age, gender, race/ethnicity, region of country)***:** Surplus sera from subjects within seven of the NHANES-III primary sampling units (PSU's) were used. These seven geographic areas were selected because they differed in their sources and treatment of drinking water. First, the PSU's were selected, then sera were selected randomly from subjects living in each PSU. Subjects included both sexes, various ages and race/ethnic subgroups.

3) **Detailed description of the goals/purpose and approach of the study:** A subset of NHANES III participants' serum was analyzed for the presence of anti- Cryptosporidium antibodies. Environmental risk factors, such as water source and preferred diet, were assessed as risk factors for seropositivity.

4) **What statistical methods and models are you using? Include a brief summary of how you present the results. If appropriate, attach sample tables and/or charts.** Univariate and Bivariate analysis were conducted. Logistic regression was used to evaluate the contribution of multiple risk factors.

5) **If you use NHANES data without publishing documents, include a brief description of these cases. (e.g., use of raw NHANES data and/or results from published NHANES studies to support setting pesticide tolerances on food, or to support setting air quality standards for ambient pollutants.): N/A**

Citation and Abstract/Executive Summary

Citation:
Hilborn E, Frost F, Neas L, Muller T, Calderon R. *Environmental Risk Factors for the presence of Cryptosporidium parvum antibodies.* Oral presentation at: International Society for Environmental Epidemiology 2000. Buffalo, New York. August, 2000.

Dates for Completed Studies:

Starting Date: **Ending Date:**

Information for Work in Progress:

Anticipated Product(s): Journal publication
Tentative Completion Date(s): December 2003

Abstract of Presentation:
Environmental Risk Factors for Presence of *Cryptosporidium parvum* Antibodies in Human Serum

E. Hilborn, F. Frost*, L. Neas, T. Muller*, R. Calderon
USEPA/HSD; *Southwest Center for Managed Care Research, Albuquerque, NM

Background - *Cryptosporidium parvum* is a parasite that infects a variety of vertebrate hosts. Sources of infection include contaminated raw produce and drinking water. Outbreaks of food borne and waterborne infections are infrequently reported, yet serological evidence suggests that infection may commonly occur.

Methods - We analyzed serum and data gathered from a convenience sample of National Health and Nutrition Examination Survey III participants to identify risk factors for the presence of anti-cryptosporidial antibodies. Seropositivity was defined as: those samples determined to contain IgG antibodies to 15/17 kDa proteins by the enzyme-linked immunoelectro-transfer blot assay with an intensity of response greater than 10% of a positive control. Data were characterized by univariate analysis. Bivariate statistical analysis and logistic regression were used to determine the association between gender, age, race, city of residence, salad and water consumption, serum carotenoids (biomarkers of exposure to produce), pet ownership, antacid and bottled water usage, home water source, and seropositivity.

Results - Of 1356 participants, 558 (41%) were seropositive. Persons resided in seven cities and ranged in age from 1-90 years (median: 38 years); 50% were female, 50% white race, 25% African-American race, and 22% Hispanic ethnicity. Seropositivity varied by city (range: 29% - 57%). Older participants were significantly more likely to be seropositive (trend $p < 0.0001$). The full regression model included gender, age, race, city, and serum alpha-carotene, all significantly associated with seropositivity; inclusion of an increased water consumption variable in the model improved the fit, but was not statistically significant ($p=0.09$). No other variables listed above were significantly associated with seropositivity.

Conclusion - These data suggest that significant differences in seropositivity exist among populations of different cities, and that prevalence of seropositivity increases with age. Increased serum alpha-carotene is significantly associated with seropositivity. Although serum alpha-carotene levels have been correlated with consumption of produce, the biomarker is not specific to the raw produce items which may be potential vehicles for oocysts. Although exposure to municipal water (by city) and serum alpha-carotene appear to be independent risk factors for seropositivity, unmeasured differences in food consumption, behavior, or cultural practices among persons living in various geographic areas may contribute to these findings. This is an abstract of a proposed presentation and does not necessarily reflect EPA policy.

Title:	Physical Activity and Nutritional Status of US Children

EPA Contact Person

Name: Thomas McCurdy   **Office Affiliation:** National Exposure Research Laboratory (NERL), Research Triangle Park, NC

Phone Number: 919-541-0782

Description of Study

1) Which NHANES did you use? ▶ **NHANES-I**   ▶ **NHANES-II**   ▶ **NHANES-III**   ☐ **HHANES** ☐ **NHANES99+** (*please check to the left of each appropriate box*)

2) **Characteristics of the study group** (*e.g., age, gender, race/ethnicity, region of country*):
Children cohorts that are defined variously by age & gender classes.

3) **Detailed description of the goals/purpose and approach of the study:**
Description of the amount of physical activity and exercise that children participate in; description of the total caloric intake of children. These data are used to evaluate the representativeness of human activity information that we use to estimate human exposure to environmental contaminants.

4) **What statistical methods and models are you using? Include a brief summary of how you present the results. If appropriate, attach sample tables and/or charts.**
Various tests of statistical hypotheses (mostly 2-sample K-S tests), analysis of variance, analysis of covariance.

5) **If you use NHANES data without publishing documents, include a brief description of these cases. (e.g., use of raw NHANES data and/or results from published NHANES studies to support setting pesticide tolerances on food, or to support setting air quality standards for ambient pollutants.):**
These analyses generally are not published, but are used for evaluating data sets that are used as inputs in in-house modeling evaluation efforts. Some of these evaluation studies will be published, but most are not.

Citation and Abstract/Executive Summary

Citation:

For Completed Studies, Provide the Following Dates:

Starting Date: **Ending Date:**

Work in Progress, Provide the Following Information:

Anticipated Product(s): Journal article on comparing exercise participation rates determined from the literature with those derived from NERL's Consolidated Human Activity Database.

Tentative Completion Date(s): FY2002

Example of the types of NHANES secondary studies that are used by this Office:

Albanes, d., Blair, A., and Taylor, P.R. (1989). "Physical activity and risk of cancer in the NHANES I population." Amer. J. Pub. Health 79: 744-750.

Blair, D., Haabicht, J.P., and Alekel, L. (1989). "Assessment of body composition, dietary patterns, and nutritional status in the National Health Examination Surveys and National Health and Nutrition Examination Surveys," pp. 79-104 in: T. Drury (ed.). Assessing Physical Fitness and Physical Activity in Population-Based Surveys. Washington DC: U.S. Government Printing Office.

Breslow, R.A., et al. (2001). "Long-term recreational physical activity and breast cancer in the National Health and Nutrition Examination Survey I epidemiologic follow-up study." Cancer Epidem. Biomark. Prev. 10: 805-808.

Briefel, R.R., McDowell, M.A., Alaimo, K., Caughman, C.R., Bischof, A.L., Carroll, M.D., and Johnson, C.L. (1995). "Total energy intake of the US population: The third National Health and Nutrition Examination Survey, 1988-1991." Amer. J. Clin. Nutr. 62(Supp.): 1072S-1080S.

Clark, G. and Whittemore, A.S. (2000). "Prostate cancer risk in relation to anthropometry and physical activity: The National Health and Nutrition Examination Survey I Epidemiological Follow-Up Study." Cancer Epidem. Biomarkers Prev. 9: 875-881.

Crespo, C.J., Smit, E., et al. (2001). "Acculturation and leisure-time physical inactivity in Mexican American adults: Results from NHANES III, 1988-1994." Amer. J. Pub. Health 91: 1254-1257.

Eck, L.H., Hackett-Renner, C., and Klesges, L.M. (1992). "Impact of diabetic status, dietary intake, physical activity, and smoking status on body mass index in NHANES II." Amer. J. Clin. Nutr. 56: 329-333.

Farmer, M.E., Locke, B.Z., Mościcki, E.K., Dannenberg, A.L., Larson, D.B., and Radloff, L.S. (1988). "Physical activity and depressive symptoms: the NHANES I epidemiologic follow-up study." Amer. J. Epidem. 128: 1340-1351.

Ford, E.S. (1998). "Characteristics of survey participants with and without a telephone: Findings from the Third National Health and Nutrition Examination Survey." J. Clin. Epidem. 51: 55-60.

Gillum, R.F., Mussolino, M.E., and Ingram, D.D. (1996). "Physical activity and stroke incidence in women and men. The NHANES I epidemiologic follow-up study." Amer. J. Epidem. 143: 860-869.

Klesges, L.M., Klesges, R.C., and Cigrang, J.A. (1992). "Discrepancies between self-reported smoking and carboxyhemoglobin: an analysis of the Second National Health and Nutrition Survey." Amer. J. Pub. Health 82: 1026-1029. McDowell, A.J. (1989). "Cardiovascular endurance, strength, and lung function tests in the National Health and Nutrition Examination Surveys," pp. 21-77 in: T. Drury (ed.). Assessing Physical Fitness and Physical Activity in Population-Based Surveys. Washington DC: U.S. Government Printing Office.

Norris, J., Harnack, L., Carmichael, S., Pouane, T., Wakimoto, P., and Block, G. (1997). "US trends in nutrient intake: the 1987 and 1992 National Health Interview Surveys." Amer. J. Pub. Health 87: 740-746.

Troiano, R.P. et al (2000). "Energy and fat intakes of children and adolescents in the United States: Data from the National Health and Nutrition Examination Surveys." Amer. J. Clin. Nutr. 72(Supp.): 1343S-1453S.

Schectman, G., McKinney, P., Pleuss, J., and Hoffman, R.G. (1990). "Dietary intake of Americans reporting adherence to a low cholesterol diet (NHANES II)." Amer. J. Public Health 80: 698-703.

Title:	Exposure Factors Handbook

EPA Contact Person

Name: Jacqueline Moya   **Office Affiliation:** National Center for Environmental Assessment (NCEA), Office of Research and Development (ORD), Washington, DC

Phone Number: 202-564-3245

Description of Study

1) Which NHANES did you use? ☐ **NHANES-I** ▶ **NHANES-II** ▶ **NHANES-III** ☐ **HHANES**
   ☐ **NHANES99+** *(check to the left of each appropriate box)*

2) **Characteristics of the study group** *(e.g., age, gender, race/ethnicity, region of country)*:
We looked at all ages and both M/F.

3) **Detailed description of the goals/purpose and approach of the study:**
To derive body weights and body surface areas based on body weight that can be used for risk and exposure assessments. The data are presented in tabular form as part of the Exposure Factors Handbook, which contains numerous tables of data on various socioeconomic and exposure-related variables derived from a variety of sources including NHANES.

4) **What statistical methods and models are you using? Include a brief summary of how you present the results. If appropriate, attach sample tables and/or charts.**
Mean and median values of body weight and body surface area were calculated for subjects by age; by gender; and by combined age and gender. Age was classified as 2-6 months, 7-12 months; then yearly until age 17; thereafter as 18-24, 25-34, 35-44, 45-54, 55-64, 65-74, 75 years and older.

5) **If you use NHANES data without publishing documents, include a brief description of these cases. (e.g., use of raw NHANES data and/or results from published NHANES studies to support setting pesticide tolerances on food, or to support setting air quality standards for ambient pollutants.):**
We used analysis done by others on the NHANES II and III data

Citation and Abstract/Executive Summary

Citation: *Exposure Factors Handbook EPA/600/P-95/002Fa-c*
Child-Specific Exposure Factors Handbook EPA/600/P/00/002F

Dates for Completed Studies:

Starting Date: **Ending Date:** EFH - 1997; CS-EFH external review draft June 2000
                                    Interim final may be released in 2002.

Information for Work in Progress:

Anticipated Product(s):
Tentative Completion Date(s):

Abstract:

The Exposure Factors Handbook provides a summary of the available statistical data on various factors used in assessing human exposure. This Handbook is addressed to exposure assessors inside the Agency as well as outside, who need to obtain data on standard factors to calculate human exposure to toxic chemicals. These factors include: drinking water consumption; soil ingestion; inhalation rates; dermal factors including skin area and soil adherence factors; consumption of fruits and vegetables, fish, meats, dairy products, homegrown foods; breast milk intake; human activity factors; consumer product use; and residential characteristics. Recommended values are for the general population and also for various segments of the population who may have characteristics different from the general population. NCEA has strived to include full discussions of the issues that assessors should consider in deciding how to use these data and recommendations. The document is in final form, but as new data become available updates will be posted on this home page.

NCEA has also produced a CD-ROM that contains an interactive version of the Exposure Factors Handbook. The CD-ROM has word search capabilities, downloadable tables, hypertext links to various chapters in the document, and key references.

A limited number of paper copies and CD-ROM version of the Handbook are available from the National Service Center for Environmental Publications (NSCEP) in Cincinnati, Ohio (phone 1-800-490-9198; 513-489-8190; fax 513-489-8695). Please provide the title and EPA number when ordering from NSCEP. Documents may also be ordered on-line at www.epa.gov/NCEPIhome/orderpub.html. Paper copies may be purchased from the National Technical Information Service (NTIS) in Springfield, VA (phone 1-800-553-NTIS[6847] or 703-605-6000; fax 703-321-8547).

Title:	The performance of human subjects on three neurobehavioral tests included in the Third National Health and Nutrition Examination Survey

EPA Contact Person

Name: David Otto   **Office Affiliation:** Clinical Research Branch, Human Studies Division (HSD), National Health & Environmental Effects Research Laboratory (NHEERL), Research Triangle Park, NC

Phone Number: (919) 966-6226

Description of Study

1) Which NHANES did you use? ☐ **NHANES-I**   ☐ **NHANES-II**   ☒ **NHANES-III**   ☐ **HHANES**
   ☐ **NHANES99+** (*check to the left of each appropriate box*)

2) Characteristics of the study group (*e.g., age, gender, race/ethnicity, region of country*)**:**
Half-sample of adults (20-59 years old) with odd-numbered survey identification numbers who participated in NHANES-III. The sample size is 5,662 and is a representative national sample. Blacks and Mexican-Americans were over-sampled to obtain more precise estimates for these groups.

3) Detailed description of the goals/purpose and approach of the study: The purpose of the study was to obtain a representative national sample of the performance of working-age adults on three computer-assisted neurobehavioral tests: simple reaction-time, symbol-digit substitution (coding) and serial digit learning (short-term memory). The tests used were from the Neurobehavioral Evaluation System (NES2). Demographic variables assessed included gender, age, educational level, family income, and race-ethnicity.

4) What statistical methods and models are you using? Include a brief summary of how you present the results. If appropriate, attach sample tables and/or charts. The sample design was a stratified, multistage probability design. Performance estimates were calculated using the NHANES-III central nervous system (CNS) sample weights (WTPFCNS6) calculated with SUDAAN (release 7.5.2). Variances were estimated by SUDAAN using a linear approximation method. Means and standard errors for performance measures are presented for gender (M/F), age groups (20-29, 30-39, 40-49, 50-59), education levels (0-8, 9-11, 12, 13+), family income (<10,000, 10,000-29,999, 30,000-49,999, >50,000) and race-ethnicity (non-Hispanic white, non-Hispanic black, Mexican American, other).

5) If you use NHANES data without publishing documents, include a brief description of these cases.   (e.g., use of raw NHANES data and/or results from published NHANES studies to support setting pesticide tolerances on food, or to support setting air quality standards for ambient pollutants.):

Citation and Abstract/Executive Summary:

Citation: Krieg, EF; Chrislip, DW; Letz, RE; Otto, DA; Crespo, CJ; Brightwell, WS; Ehrenberg, RL. The performance of human subjects on three neurobehavioral tests included in the Third National Health and Nutrition Examination Survey. *Neurotoxicology and Teratology* (2001), 23:569-589.

Dates for Completed Studies:

Starting Date: 1988   **Ending Date:** 1994

Information for Work in Progress:

Anticipated Product(s):
Tentative Completion Date(s): NA

Abstract:

KRIEG, JR., E. F., D. W. CHRISLIP, R. E. LETZ, D. A. OTTO, C. J. CRESPO, W. S. BRIGHTWELL AND R. L. EHRENBERG. *Neurobehavioral Test Performance in the third National Health and Nutrition Examination Survey.* NEUROTOXICOL TERATOL (2001), 23:569-589. The third National Health and Nutrition Examination Survey (NHANES III) contained three computerized neurobehavioral tests from the Neurobehavioral Evaluation System: simple reaction time, symbol-digit substitution, and serial digit learning. The neurobehavioral data that were collected came from a nationally representative sample of adults 20 to 59 years old. Performance on the tests was related to sex, age, education level, family income, and race-ethnicity. Performance decreased as age increased, and increased as education level and family income increased. Differences in performance between sexes, levels of education, and racial-ethnic groups tended to decrease as family income increased. The relationship between age and performance on the symbol-digit substitution test varied by education level and by racial-ethnic group. The relationship between age and performance on the serial digit learning test varied by racial-ethnic group. Questionnaire variables that were related to performance on one or more of the tests included the reported amount of last night's sleep, energy level, computer or video game familiarity, alcoholic beverages within the last three hours, and effort. Persons who took the tests in English or Spanish performed differently on the symbol-digit substitution and serial digit learning tests. Performance on all the tests decreased as test room temperature increased.

Title:	Examination of Risk Factors for Respiratory Effects in Children: Use of NHANES-III Respiratory Health and EPA Air Monitoring Data. Part IV: Estimation of Ambient Air Pollutant Concentrations and Their Effects on Children's Respiratory Health

EPA Contact Person

Name: Susan Perlin	Office Affiliation: National Center for Environmental Assessment (NCEA); Office of Research and Development (ORD), Washington, DC
Phone Number:202-564-3248	

Description of Study

1) Which NHANES did you use? ☐ NHANES-I ☐ NHANES-II ☒ NHANES-III ☐ HHANES
☐ NHANES99+ (*please check to the left of each appropriate box*)

2) Characteristics of the study group (*e.g., age, gender, race/ethnicity, region of country*)**:** All children and adolescents 0-16 years of age. This is a data set of 13,944 subjects and includes both sexes and all ethnic groups. In these children, we evaluate outdoor and indoor environmental effects on asthma prevalence, respiratory symptom prevalence, and spirometric lung function (e.g., FVC, FEV_1). NHANES-III collected data on asthma and respiratory symptoms for all children, regardless of age, but performed lung function tests only on subjects 8 years and older.

3) Detailed description of the goals/purpose and approach of the study: This is a multi-part study to evaluate risk factors for respiratory effects (i.e., lung function and symptomatology) in children. Parts 1-3 are described in preceding project summaries (Contact Person: Robert Chapman) and address risk factors based only on data collected in NHANES-III. The remainder of the work builds on models developed in Parts 1-3 to examine risk factors associated with ambient air quality and urbanization. Geographic information system (GIS) technology is used with non-NHANES databases to develop measures of ambient air pollution, population density and road density for each year of the Survey for all locations with NHANES-III subjects. Environmental variables are estimated at the census block group level (BG) and linked at that level to the NHANES-III subjects. To maintain subject confidentiality, the National Center for Health Statistics does all the data linking and runs all models on the linked data. EPA's national air monitoring data are used to estimate levels of atmospheric pollution (O3, PM10, SOx, NOx, CO and Pb). Monitoring data are interpolated to estimate ambient air pollutant concentrations for all BGs in the NHANES-III counties. As yet, there is no scientific consensus as to the interpolation method of choice. Therefore, so several different interpolation methods are used to derive air concentration levels and determine the conditions under which different methods produce significantly different concentration values. Method-specific concentration values are linked with each NHANES-III subject to ascertain and compare the impact of alternative methodologic approaches on the evaluation of environmental health effects.

4) What statistical methods and models are you using? Include a brief summary of how you present the results. If appropriate, attach sample tables and/or charts. Kriging, spatial averaging, nearest neighbor and inverse distance weighting are the interpolation methods used to estimate concentration levels of pollutants (O3, PM10, SOx, NOx, CO and Pb) at the BG level for NHANES-III counties. Population density is calculated from 1990 census data by dividing the total population by the land area for each BG. A measure of road density has tentatively been calculated using 1990 Census TIGER data and estimating the length of road segments for each BG.
Regression models developed in Parts 1-3 of this study incorporate variables such as active and passive smoking, presence of home combustion devices, allergy status of subjects, parental history of asthma and allergies, and socioeconomic and demographic characteristics of subjects and their families to determine their effects on respiratory health of children. As a starting point, interpolated air concentration values, other measures of urbanization, and meteorologic variables will be added to these regression models to evaluate the impact of ambient environmental exposures on children's respiratory health.

5) If you use NHANES data without publishing documents, include a brief description of these cases. (e.g., use of raw NHANES data and/or results from published NHANES studies to support setting pesticide tolerances on food, or to support setting air quality standards for ambient pollutants.):

Citation:

Starting Date:	**Ending Date:**

Anticipated Product(s):
1) EPA report "Examination of Risk Factors for Respiratory Effects in Children: Use of NHANES-III Respiratory Health and EPA Air Monitoring Data" (tentative title) describes the four interpolation methods and results across all BGs in all NHANES-III counties for O3 and PM10 for the year 1990.

2) Several journal articles to be written for publication detailing evaluation of the linked health and exposure data.

Tentative Completion Date(s):
1) EPA report: External review of draft report completed. Finalized report should be completed by 3/02.

2) Journal articles will be written and submitted for publication during 2002 - 2004.

Title:	Development of Methods, Data, and a Model of Human Cumulative Exposure, Dose, and Health Risks for Pyrethroid Insecticides – Task 4: Evaluation of dietary exposure model

EPA Contact Person

Name: James Quackenboss   **Office Affiliation:** National Exposure Research Laboratory (NERL), Human Exposure & Atmospheric Sciences Division, Office of Research and Development (ORD), Las Vegas, NV

Phone Number: (702) 798-2442

Description of Study

1) Which NHANES did you use? ☐ NHANES-I ☐ NHANES-II ☐ NHANES-III ☐ HHANES ☑ NHANES99+
(*check to the left of each appropriate box*)

2) Characteristics of the study group (*e.g., age, gender, race/ethnicity, region of country*)**:** Sample of adults and children whose urine samples were analyzed for pesticide metabolites, and who provided food diaries.

3) Detailed description of the goals/purpose and approach of the study: The objective of the overall study is to develop an exposure-dose-response model that will allow for more well-informed decisions on managing the potential cumulative risks associated with aggregate exposures to pyrethroids. The purpose of this task is to evaluate a dietary exposure model which is based on individual food consumption patterns collected in NHANES 99+ and currently available food residue databases.

Approach: Estimates of the subjects' dietary exposure to several pyrethroids will be modeled using their food diaries and information on food pesticide residues. A dose-estimating model will then be used to derive the corresponding urine-metabolite concentrations. These urine-metabolite estimates will be compared with the subjects' urine-metabolite concentrations measured in NHANES99+ to provide a "reality check" on indirect estimates of dietary exposure, and to identify the relative contribution of dietary exposure to the total eliminated dose. The SHEDS (Stochastic Human Exposure and Dose Simulation) model dietary module currently uses the 1994-96 and 1998 Continuing Survey of Food Intake by Individuals (CSFII) consumption data, and available food pesticide residue databases, including USDA's Pesticide Data Program (PDP) and FDA's Total Diet Study (TDS). SHEDS will be adapted to use food consumption records for the same individuals who have urine-metabolite results in NHANES99+. The metabolite currently available for NHANES99+, 3-phenoxybenzoic acid (3PBA), is the common metabolite of several pyrethroids including permethrin, cypermethrin, deltamethrin, tralomethrin, fenvalerate, cyhalothrin, fluvalinate, and esfenvalerate. Multiple simulations will be conducted for each individual's consumption record to characterize both variability and uncertainty in the exposure estimates. (SHEDS uses a two-stage Monte Carlo approach to estimate uncertainty distributions). Within-individual variability will include differences in residue concentrations. Model uncertainties include assumptions made for food items and pesticides not represented in the available residue databases, differences between food consumption and residue databases (e.g., relating CSFII consumption information to pesticide concentrations for TDS foods), and methods for handling observations below the detection limits. The Exposure Related Dose Estimating Model (ERDEM) will use published PK parameters, together with absorption and elimination coefficients determined in this Project (Task 1), to estimate blood and urine-metabolite concentrations.

4) What statistical methods and models are you using? Include a brief summary of how you present the results. If appropriate, attach sample tables and/or charts.
A distribution of metabolite concentrations will be calculated for each individual. The 95%-confidence intervals for the individual's mean will be compared with the urine-metabolite concentration measured by CDC for the NHANES 99+. This comparison will be grouped by residential insecticide usage during the previous month, as reported in the NHANES Pesticide Use Questionnaire, to help distinguish dietary from other sources of these exposures.

The measured metabolite concentrations provide an upper limit for defining acceptable model performance. Thus, if the model is performing adequately then we should expect dietary exposure to account for some percentage (<100%) of the measured urine-metabolite concentrations, plus or minus the variability and uncertainty bounds. The remaining excreted dose provides an estimate of the contribution from non-dietary exposures that are present in the US population.

5) If you use NHANES data without publishing documents, include a brief description of these cases. (e.g., use of raw NHANES data and/or results from published NHANES studies to support setting pesticide tolerances on food, or to support setting air quality standards for ambient pollutants.):

This task is part of a proposal which was submitted in response to a "Call for Pre-Proposals for Collaborative Research on Intermittent Exposure/Risk in Support of ORD Safe Food Research Program." The project was approved in 1/02.

Citation:

Starting Date:	Ending Date:

Anticipated Product(s): manuscript on comparison of SHEDS-ERDEM (exposure-dose) model with pesticide metabolites
Tentative Completion Date(s): Task 4 is planned for FY2003; the manuscript will be prepared in FY04

Title:	Hispanic Health and Nutrition Examination Survey (HHANES), 1982-1984. Pesticides in urine and blood.

EPA Contact Person

Name: Dina M. Schreinemachers   **Office Affiliation:** Epidemiology and Biomarkers Branch, Human Studies Division (HSD), National Health & Environmental Effects Research Laboratory (NHEERL), Research Triangle Park, NC

Phone Number: (919) 966-5875

Description of Study

1) Which NHANES did you use? ☐ NHANES-I   ☐ NHANES-II   ☐ NHANES-III   ▣ HHANES
  ☐ NHANES99+ *(check to the left of each appropriate box)*

2) Characteristics of the study group *(e.g., age, gender, race/ethnicity, region of country)*:
HHANES (1982 - 1984) examined three distinct U.S. Hispanic subpopulations: Mexican-Americans living in CA, AZ, NM, CO, and TX; Cuban-Americans living in Dade county, FL; and Puerto Ricans living in the New York City area. We studied both men and women, ages 12-74, for these three subpopulations.

3) Detailed description of the goals/purpose and approach of the study:
Report on pesticide residue and metabolite levels in the blood of all 3 Hispanic subpopulations and the urine of the Mexican-Americans.

4) What statistical methods and models are you using? Include a brief summary of how you present the results. If appropriate, attach sample tables and/or charts.
 Means and frequencies of pesticide residues and metabolites. Pesticide levels in this report are determined by gender for children aged 12-17, and adults aged 18-74. The percentage of subjects and estimated population at or above the level of detection, and the percentile distributions are determined for each pesticide residue. The pesticide and metabolite data themselves should not be interpreted in relation to one another (e.g., the ratio of metabolites to a specific compound to each other), since no individual data are provided in this report. The proportion of exposed people and the average exposure levels can be compared across populations.

5) If you use NHANES data without publishing documents, include a brief description of these cases.   (e.g., use of raw NHANES data and/or results from published NHANES studies to support setting pesticide tolerances on food, or to support setting air quality standards for ambient pollutants.):

Citation and Abstract/Executive Summary

Citation: Schreinemachers DM, Gonzales M, Everson RB, Mendola P, Ray BM, Lewis DR. Hispanic Health and Nutrition Examination Survey, 1982-1984. Pesticides in urine and blood. EPA Report, in press.

Dates for Completed Studies:

Starting Date: 1998   **Ending Date:** 2000

Information for Work in Progress:

Anticipated Product(s):
Tentative Completion Date(s):

Abstract:
    The Hispanic Health and Nutrition Examination Survey, conducted during 1982 - 1984 by the National Center for Health Statistics, examined the nutritional and health status of three distinct U.S. Hispanic subpopulations: Mexican-Americans living in California, Arizona, New Mexico, Colorado, and Texas; Cuban-Americans living in Dade county, Florida; and Puerto Ricans living in the New York City area.

The Environmental Protection Agency sponsored the measurement of pesticide residues and metabolites in serum for a subset of each of the three subpopulations, and in urine for a subset only of the Mexican-Americans. The following pesticides were included in the analyses: urinary malathion metabolites (malathion mono- and dicarboxylic acid); urinary multiphenols (2,4-dichloro phenoxy acetic acid, dicamba, para-nitrophenol, pentachlorophenol, 2,4,5-trichloro phenoxy acetic acid, 2,4,5-trichlorophenol, Silvex, 3,5,6-trichloro-2-pyridinol); and serum chlorinated pesticides (aldrin; α-, β-, γ-, and δ-hexachlorocyclohexane, o,p'-DDD, p,p'-DDD, op'-DDE, pp'-DDE, op'-DDT, pp'-DDT, dieldrin, endrin, heptachlor epoxide, heptachlor, hexachlorobenzene, mirex, oxychlordane, polychlorinated biphenyls, trans-nonachlor). Laboratory methods for the pesticide analyses included flame photometric chromatography for the malathion urinary metabolites, and electron capture gas chromatography for both the urinary multiphenols and chlorinated pesticides in serum. Laboratory methods and QA/QC procedures are described in detail.

This report presents the percent of subjects with quantifiable levels of the pesticides residues and metabolites and their distribution percentiles for two age groups (12-17, 18-74), by gender and subpopulation. For each pesticide, use, route of exposure, and potential health effects are discussed. These data provide an estimate of the general prevalence of exposure in these three Hispanic subpopulations, and will contribute to studies involving comparison of the general U.S. population and the Hispanic-American subpopulations.

Title:	Aspirin use and lung, colon, and breast cancer incidence in a prospective study

EPA Contact Person

Name: Dina M. Schreinemachers **Office Affiliation:** Epidemiology and Biomarkers Branch, Human Studies Division (HSD), National Health & Environmental Effects Research Laboratory (NHEERL), Research Triangle Park, NC

Phone Number: (919) 966-5875

Description of Study

1) Which NHANES did you use? ☒ **NHANES-I**   ☐ **NHANES-II** ☐ **NHANES-III** ☐ **HHANES**   ☐ **NHANES99+**
(please check to the left of each appropriate box)
We used NHANES-I including the follow-up survey

2) Characteristics of the study group *(e.g., age, gender, race/ethnicity, region of country)*:
Men and women, white and nonwhite, USA., ages 25-74

3) Detailed description of the goals/purpose and approach of the study:
Study the of association between aspirin use and cancer risk

4) What statistical methods and models are you using? Include a brief summary of how you present the results. If appropriate, attach sample tables and/or charts.
Mantel-Haenszel analyses and proportional hazards models

5) If you use NHANES data without publishing documents, include a brief description of these cases.   (e.g., use of raw NHANES data and/or results from published NHANES studies to support setting pesticide tolerances on food, or to support setting air quality standards for ambient pollutants.):

Citation and Abstract/Executive Summary

Citation:
Schreinemachers DM, Everson RB. Aspirin use and lung, colon, and breast cancer incidence in a prospective study. Epidemiology 5: 138-146, 1994.

For Completed Studies, Provide the Following Dates:

Starting Date: 1992   **Ending Date:** 1994

Work in Progress, Provide the Following Information:

Anticipated Product(s):
Tentative Completion Date(s):

Abstract:
A large body of experimental data and several recent epidemiologic studies suggest that aspirin use may decrease cancer risk. The experimental studies found effects at many anatomic sites, while the epidemiologic studies saw the greatest effect on mortality from digestive cancers. To provide further human data, we examined the association between aspirin use and cancer risk using data from the National Health and Nutrition Examination Survey I (NHANES I) and the NHANES I Epidemiologic Followup Studies (NHEFS). Characterization of aspirin use was based on questions in the baseline interview asking whether subjects used aspirin during the previous 30 days. Data were available from 12,668 subjects aged 25-74 at time of initial examination for NHANES I, who were followed for an average of 12.4 years. Among these subjects 1,257 were diagnosed with cancer more than two years after their NHANES I exam. Incidence of several cancers was lower among persons who reported aspirin use: the incidence rate ratio and 95% CI for all sites combined were 0.83 [0.74-0.93], lung cancer 0.68 [0.49-0.94], breast cancer in women 0.70 [0.50-0.96], and colorectal cancer in younger men 0.35 [0.17-0.73]. These findings were not readily

explained by potentially confounding factors. The data suggest an association between aspirin consumption and decreased cancer incidence at several cancer sites.

Title:	Risk Assessment for Toxic Substances Control Act, Section 403, Lead Standards

EPA Contact Person

Name: Brad Schultz and Ron Morony

Office Affiliation: Office of Pollution, Prevention and Toxics (OPPT), National Program Chemicals Div. (NPCD), Office of Prevention, Pesticides and Toxic Substances (OPPTS), Washington, DC

Phone Number: 202-260-3896 (Brad) 202-260-0282 (Ron)

Description of Study

1) Which NHANES did you use? ☐ NHANES-I ☐ NHANES-II ☒ NHANES-III ☐ HHANES
☐ **NHANES99+** *(check to the left of each appropriate box)*

2) Characteristics of the study group *(e.g., age, gender, race/ethnicity, region of country)*:
We used the nationally representative sample of children 1-5 years of age, and also looked at subgroups separately by race, age of housing, and economic status.

3) Detailed description of the goals/purpose and approach of the study:
We used the blood lead (PbB) level data to establish a baseline for lead exposure in children ages 1-5 years. This baseline represents the level of risk to this subgroup before there are any reductions in exposures due to the promulgation of new lead exposure standards in dust, soil, and paint.

4) What statistical methods and models are you using? Include a brief summary of how you present the results. If appropriate, attach sample tables and/or charts.
PbB data, adjusted by NHANES sampling weights, was used as input to risk models linking blood-lead levels with health effects. The models link PbB levels to IQ deficits as described in the two reports below. Also, lognormal distribution of PbB levels were used, as appropriate, as an approximation for the purpose of making presentations.

5) If you use NHANES data without publishing documents, include a brief description of these cases. (e.g., use of raw NHANES data and/or results from published NHANES studies to support setting pesticide tolerances on food, or to support setting air quality standards for ambient pollutants.):
Not applicable.

Citation and Abstract/Executive Summary

Citations:
Risk Analysis to Support Standards for Lead in Paint, Dust, and Soil (EPA 747-R-97-006), June 1998.
Full Report Available at http://www.epa.gov/lead/403risk.htm
Executive Summary available at http://www.epa.gov/lead/raexsumm.pdf

Risk Analysis to Support Standards for Lead in Paint, Dust, and Soil: Supplemental Report (EPA 747-R-00-004), December 2000
Full Report Available at http://www.epa.gov/lead/403risksupp.htm
Executive Summary Available at http://www.epa.gov/lead/rasuppexsumm.pdf

Dates for Completed Studies:

Starting Date: 1992   **Ending Date:** December 2000

Information for Work in Progress:

Anticipated Product(s):
Tentative Completion Date(s):

Abstract:

Risk Analysis to Support Standards for Lead in Paint, Dust, and Soil:

Lead poisoning in children is recognized as a major health problem in the United States. While there are many sources of lead in the human environment, lead-based paint hazards in residential housing are considered the primary source of lead exposure for children. To help develop a national strategy to eliminate lead-based paint hazards, the President of the United States signed into law the Residential Lead-Based Paint Hazard Reduction Act of 1992 (42 U.S.C. 4851). This legislation included an amendment to the Toxic Substances Control Act (Title

IV: Lead Exposure Reduction), requiring the Administrator of the U.S. Environmental Protection Agency (EPA) to enact a variety of activities to identify and reduce environmental exposure to lead hazards. Specifically, §403 of TSCA (15 U.S.C. 2683) states: "... the Administrator shall promulgate regulations which shall identify, for purposes of this title and the Residential Lead-Based Paint Hazard Reduction Act of 1992, lead-based paint hazards, lead-contaminated dust, and lead-contaminated soil."

Under §403, the Agency is required to identify what constitutes a lead-based paint hazard (i.e., conditions that cause exposure to lead-contaminated dust, soil, or paint that would result in adverse health effects to humans) and what constitutes lead contamination of dust and soil (i.e., the presence of lead levels which can pose a threat of adverse health effects). In particular, the §403 rule to be established by the Agency will set standards for lead levels in dust and soil to determine 1) whether a residential environment has lead-contaminated dust and soil, and 2) whether a lead-based paint hazard is present in a residential environment.

This report presents the methods and findings of a risk analysis, which provides a scientific foundation for the regulatory standards that the Agency will establish in response to §403. This risk analysis consists of two parts. Part I (Chapters 2 through 5) constitutes the risk assessment, or EPA's assessment of the health risks to young children from exposures to lead-based paint hazards, lead-contaminated dust, and lead-contaminated soil in the nation's housing. Part II (Chapter 6) constitutes an analysis of risk management options, which includes the Agency's approach to estimating how these risks are reduced following promulgation of the §403 rule and illustrates use of this methodology for a broad range of example options for the §403 standards. The objective of the risk assessment is to characterize *baseline* health risks to young children from specific residential exposures to lead. The term *baseline* (or "pre-§403") refers to conditions in 1997, prior to promulgating any rule in response to §403. The objectives of risk management are to develop and apply methodology to determine how risks are expected to be reduced from baseline levels because of interventions conducted in response to the §403 rule (or "post §403"), and to develop an approach to estimate numbers of children and housing units that would be directly impacted by the rule. Information presented in this risk analysis will ultimately be used to consider various standards for rulemaking and as input to the Regulatory Impacts Analysis (RIA) for the proposed rule, as well as any interim economic cost-benefit analyses.

Title:	The Decline in Blood Lead Levels in Children 1-5 Years of Age

EPA Contact Person

Name: John Schwemberger   **Office Affiliation:** Office of Pollution, Prevention and Toxics (OPPT), National Program Chemicals Div. (NPCD), Office of Prevention, Pesticides and Toxic Substances (OPPTS), Washington, DC

Phone Number: 202-260-7195

Description of Study

1) Which NHANES did you use? ☐ NHANES-I   ▶ NHANES-II   ▶ NHANES-III   ☐ HHANES
☐ NHANES99+ *(check to the left of each appropriate box)*

2) Characteristics of the study group *(e.g., age, gender, race/ethnicity, region of country)*:
The study group was children 1 to 5 years old.

3) Detailed description of the goals/purpose and approach of the study:
The goal of the study was to develop a graph showing the decline in children's blood lead (PbB) levels over time and to compare the graph with time points when federal actions designed to lower exposure to lead went into effect.

4) What statistical methods and models are you using? Include a brief summary of how you present the results. If appropriate, attach sample tables and/or charts.
Geometric mean (µg/dl) of PbB calculated for children ages 1-5 years either for a year or for a three year period in the case of NHANES III.

5) If you use NHANES data without publishing documents, include a brief description of these cases.   (e.g., use of raw NHANES data and/or results from published NHANES studies to support setting pesticide tolerances on food, or to support setting air quality standards for ambient pollutants.):
Not applicable.

Citation and Abstract/Executive Summary

Citations:
Goldman, LR, Linking Research and Policy to Ensure Children's Environmental Health, **Environmental Health Perspectives** 106 (Supplement 3), 1998, pp. 857-862. Available at:
http://ehpnet1.niehs.nih.gov/members/1998/Suppl-3/857-862goldman/goldman-full.html

Office of Pollution Prevention and Toxics Program Activities for Fiscal Years 1998 and 1999, (EPA 745-K-99-003), December 1999, p. 19. Available at http://www.epa.gov/oppt/ar98-99/opptreport.pdf.

Dates for Completed Studies:

Starting Date: 1997   **Ending Date:** 1998 (Goldman Article), 1999 (OPPT Report)

Information for Work in Progress:

Anticipated Product(s): Graph will be updated when NHANES 2000 and 2001 blood lead statistics are available.
Tentative Completion Date(s): April 2001 and April 2002

Abstract from Goldman et al, 1998:
Prevention of Childhood Lead Exposure
Blood lead levels previously considered safe are now known to be associated with adverse health effects in children. Since 1970, the level of concern for blood lead has been revised downward, from 60 to 10 µµg/dl. Research with more sensitive measures

and better study designs demonstrated that the level of concern for childhood lead poisoning should be lowered. This research was largely supported by the federal government, especially the NIEHS, the CDC, and the U.S. EPA.

Over this same time span from 1970 to the present, a number of federal policy actions were taken to reduce exposures to lead. These actions include several laws and standards: the 1971 Lead-Based Paint Poisoning Prevention Act (*17*); the U.S. EPA phase out of lead in gasoline starting in 1973 (*18*) with completion at the end of 1995 (*19*); the U.S. EPA ban on use of lead in plumbing, fixtures, fittings, and solder (*20*); the U.S. Consumer Product Safety Commission 1978 standard limiting the allowable amount of lead in paint (*21*); the reduction and elimination of the lead in solder for food cans in the United States, with the final U.S. FDA rule effective in December 1995 (*22*); the Residential Lead-Based Paint Hazard Reduction Act of 1992 (*23*) (generally referred to as Title X), which mandated additional actions by the U.S. EPA, the U.S. Department of Housing and Urban Development (HUD), and other federal agencies. Title X requirements involving the U.S. EPA include new efforts on education; training and certification/standards for abatement activities; real estate notification (giving the public the right to know about the presence of lead in a home before buying or renting it); and development of lead-contaminated soil and dust standards (*23*). Much of this work has been accomplished, but there is still much to do. The U.S. EPA must develop lead-contaminated soil and dust standards. States need to adopt abatement programs. Important strides have been made through education, but the sources of lead hazards must be removed from children's environments.

Measures to prevent and reduce childhood lead poisoning have paid great dividends (Figure 1). According to the most recent report from the CDC, NHANES III, data show the rate of lead poisoning has been halved since the beginning of this decade and continues the downward trend observed since the late 1970s (*24*). At that time, the average blood lead level in children 1 to 5 years of age was 15 μμg/dl. Average blood lead levels today are 2.7 μμg/dl. In the late 1970s almost 88% of children 1 to 5 years of age had elevated blood lead levels, compared to approximately 4.4% of children today.

Figure 1. Chronological trend in blood lead levels for U.S. children 1 to 5 years of age and regulatory actions taken to reduce lead exposure to children, 1971 to 1995. Federal actions: *1*) 1971, Lead-Based Paint Poisoning Prevention Act (*17*); *2*) 1973, U.S. EPA begins phase out of lead in gasoline (*18*); *3*) 1978, U.S. Consumer Product Safety Commission bans sale and distribution of lead-based paint (*21*); *4*) 1986, lead in plumbing, fixtures, fittings, and solder banned (*20*); *5*) 1992, Lead Title X to abate lead hazards in housing (*23*); *6*) 1995, U.S. EPA completes phase out of leaded gasoline (*19*).

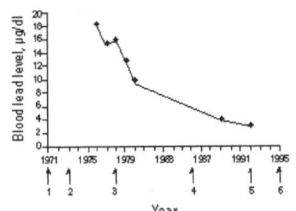

Title:	Variability in Puberty Measures in Children in Response to Classes of Chemicals-NHANES-III

EPA Contact Person

Name: Sherry Selevan   **Office Affiliation**: National Center for Environmental Assessment (NCEA-W), Office of Research and Development (ORD), Washington, DC

Phone Number: 202-564-3403

Description of Study

1) Which NHANES did you use? ☐ NHANES-I   ☐ NHANES-II   ☒ NHANES-III   ☐ HHANES   ☐ NHANES99+ (*check to the left of each appropriate box*)

2) Characteristics of the study group (*e.g., age, gender, race/ethnicity, region of country*):

8-18 year olds; male and female; non-Hispanic whites, non-Hispanic blacks, Mexican-Americans; all regions

3) Detailed description of the goals/purpose and approach of the study:

To provide an overview of the variability in response of children to exposure to certain classes of chemicals using NHANES-III data. The study examines the effects of these classes of chemicals on timing of puberty onset in adolescent males and females, and the variability of response based on age, race, sex, and socioeconomic status (SES). Measures of timing of puberty available in NHANES-III include Tanner stages for pubic hair development and breast development, and age at onset of menarche. Assessment of the variability in these responses includes evaluating the proportion of individuals who have the effect or event (for example, a particular Tanner stage) for a particular exposure, the average age of each event, and the impact of the identified exposures on the average ages for these events. The exposure information available in NHANES-III falls into 2 primary categories: those measured clinically (e.g., serum levels of lead, cadmium, cotinine), and information recalled by subjects via questionnaire (e.g., active and passive smoking).

4) What statistical methods and models are you using? Include a brief summary of how you present the results. If appropriate, attach sample tables and/or charts.

All analyses include the sampling weights addressing the complex multilevel design of NHANES-III, through the use of SUDAAN.

Statistical methods include descriptive statistics (means for measurements and ages, proportions for dichotomous data such as "ever smoked, yes/no") and significance testing for differences in the descriptive statistics between demographic groups.

Statistical models allowing for consideration of related influences (such as body weight) or simultaneous, confounding exposures (for which data are available in NHANES-III) include proportional hazards analysis for time-related outcomes, and ordinal logistic regression for categorical outcomes (i.e., Tanner stage attainment at specific ages).

5) If you use NHANES data without publishing documents, include a brief description of these cases. (e.g., use of raw NHANES data and/or results from published NHANES studies to support setting pesticide tolerances on food, or to support setting air quality standards for ambient pollutants.):

Not applicable.

Citation:

Starting Date:	Ending Date:

Anticipated Product(s): Currently anticipate at least 3 reports:

1. Environment and Puberty in Girls: Examination of association of pubertal timing with blood lead and passive smoking data in the National Health and Nutrition Examination Survey III - report to satisfy Annual Performance Measure (APM)# 149

2. An examination of puberty in girls and the remaining exposures measured in NHANES-III

3. At least one report studying the above associations in boys aged 8-18 years

Tentative Completion Date(s):

1. December 2001, currently under NCEA management clearance process

2. FY2002

3. FY2003

Title:	Blood Lead Concentrations of U.S. Adult Females: Summary Statistics from Phases 1 and 2 of the National Health and Nutrition Evaluation Survey (NHANES III)

EPA Contact Person

Name: Marc Stifelman   **Office Affiliation**: Office of Environmental Assessment, EPA Region 10, Seattle, WA.

Phone Number: (206) 553-6979

Description of Study

1) Which NHANES did you use? ☐ NHANES-I   ☐ NHANES-II ▣ NHANES-III ☐ HHANES   ☐ NHANES99+
(*check to the left of each appropriate box*)

2) Characteristics of the study group (*e.g., age, gender, race/ethnicity, region of country*)**:**

Females, 17-45 years old analyzed together and by race/ethnicity and region of country.

3) Detailed description of the goals/purpose and approach of the study:

The purpose of the study was to re-evaluate default values for the geometric mean (GM) and geometric standard deviation (GSD) of blood lead (PbB) concentration that are used in the Adult Lead Methodology (ALM). Previous estimates were based on NHANES III, Phase 1 only; this analysis used Phases 1 and 2 of NHANES III.

4) What statistical methods and models are you using? Include a brief summary of how you present the results. If appropriate, attach sample tables and/or charts. SAS was used to estimate the GM and GSD for PbB for the entire US population of non-institutionalized females, 17-45 years old, and for subgroups of the population that were stratified by the race and geographic regions provided in NHANES III. Standard errors were reported for the GM using SUDAAN and the sample weights provided in NHANES III. When estimating a measure of variability, such as the GSD, the sample weights provided in NHANES III do not fully account for the complex sampling design used in NHANES III. To partially address the uncertainty in the estimates of GSD obtained from SAS, the GSD was also estimated from lognormal probability plots fit to percentiles estimated from the data. Estimates from the two methods compare favorably, with a mean difference of 0.10µg/dl. The sensitivity of the parameter estimates to the treatment of non-detects is also addressed.

Parameter estimates are provided in a series of tables for the population as a whole as well as by subgroups (i.e., race/ethnicity and geographic region); the probability plots are also provided. Percentiles of the distribution of PbB are provided, with their standard errors and 90% confidence intervals. The effect of the recommended updated parameter values on preliminary remediation goals calculated from the ALM are presented in a table.

Estimates of the GM and GSD for Mexican-Americans in the northeast region were highly uncertain due to the small sample size (24).

5) If you use NHANES data without publishing documents, include a brief description of these cases.   (e.g., use of raw NHANES data and/or results from published NHANES studies to support setting pesticide tolerances on food, or to support setting air quality standards for ambient pollutants.):

Citation and Abstract/Executive Summary

Citation:

Dates for Completed Studies:

Starting Date: **Ending Date:**

Information for Work in Progress:

Anticipated Product(s): Technical Support Document (http://www.epa.gov/superfund/programs/lead/prods.htm)

Tentative Completion Date(s): November, 2001

Title:	Sociodemographic Data For Use In Identifying Potentially Highly Exposed Children's Populations

EPA Contact Person

Name: Amina Wilkins   **Office Affiliation:** National Center for Environmental Assessment (NCEA), Office of Research and Development (ORD), Washington, DC

Phone Number: 202 564-3256

Description of Study

1) Which NHANES did you use? ☐ NHANES-I   ☐ NHANES-II   ☒ NHANES-III   ☐ HHANES   ☐ NHANES99+
(*check to the left of each appropriate box*)

2) Characteristics of the study group *(e.g., age, gender, race/ethnicity, region of country)*:

Children and adolescents ages 1-19 years of age from Phase 2 of NHANES-III, which was conducted 1991-1994. We looked at many variables, including body weight, blood lead levels (PbB), race/ethnicity, housing characteristics, and various demographic and socioeconomic characteristics.

3) Detailed description of the goals/purpose and approach of the study:

Derive the distribution of overweight children and adolescents (ages 6-17 years old) by gender, race, and age. Also derive the distribution of children and adolescents (1-19 years old) with PbB levels >10μg/dl by age, gender, race/ethnicity, housing characteristics, income and urban-rural status. These data can be used for risk and exposure assessments and will be presented in tabular form as part of a guidance document, *Sociodemographic Data For Use In Identifying Potentially Highly Exposed Children's Populations*. This document will contain numerous tables of data on various socioeconomic and exposure-related variables relevant to children and adolescents and derived from a variety of sources including NHANES.

4) What statistical methods and models are you using? Include a brief summary of how you present the results. If appropriate, attach sample tables and/or charts.

Data are presented as simple distributions of overweight individuals and individuals with PbB levels >10μg/dl by age, race, etc.

5) If you use NHANES data without publishing documents, include a brief description of these cases.   (e.g., use of raw NHANES data and/or results from published NHANES studies to support setting pesticide tolerances on food, or to support setting air quality standards for ambient pollutants.):

Citation and Abstract/Executive Summary:

Citation:

Dates for Completed Studies:

Starting Date: **Ending Date:**

Information for Work in Progress:

Anticipated Product(s): EPA guidance document, *Sociodemographic Data Used For Identifying Potentially Highly Exposed Children's Populations*, and possible website/weblinks.

Tentative Completion Date(s): 2005

Abstract:

The specific goals of the document *Sociodemographic Data for Use in Identifying Potentially Highly Exposed Children's Populations* will be to (1) help assessors identify potentially highly exposed children's populations and (2) help assessors estimate the size of these populations. It will provide information, when available, on the number of individuals, or the percent of the general population, associated with dietary preferences, cultural practices, geographic location and setting (i.e., urban vs. rural), and other activities that target populations and individuals as being possibly highly exposed. Data will be presented as they appear in the original studies/reports. Research on children's exposures/risks due to environmental contaminants has been minimal prior to the mid-1990s (before the Executive Order on the Protection of children from Environmental Risks and safety Risks, was signed on April 21, 1997). Thus the literature summaries to be provided will not be all inclusive, but will be meant to provide the reader with a general overview of available children's population data. In most cases, data will be from government publications, peer-reviewed literature, and trade associations.

The *Sociodemographic Data* document is intended to be used in conjunction with the *Child-Specific Exposure Factors Handbook* currently being developed. The *Handbook* will provide statistical data on human characteristics and behaviors (e.g., ingestion rates of foods, activity duration and frequency, soil ingestion rates, body weight, skin surface area) used in assessing exposure. Where possible, data for specific ages, gender, and race/ethnic groups will be presented. The procedure for using these two documents in combination will be as follows:

• Use the *Sociodemographic Data* document to help determine if potentially highly exposed populations may exist in the area of interest and to estimate the number of children of concern.

• Identify the suspected potentially highly exposed populations, then use the *Child-Specific Exposure Factors Handbook* to select the exposure factor values specific to the population of interest. These exposure factor values would then be combined with site-specific information on environmental contaminant concentrations to estimate exposure levels.

REFERENCES

NHANES Consortium Meeting, 2002. NCHS conducts a Consortium meeting once or twice a year for all the federal agencies to update them on the status of the survey in the field. This meeting was held at NCHS headquarters in Hyattsville, MD on February 28.

NCHS (National Center for Health Statistics), 1973. *Plan and Operation of the Health and Nutrition Examination Survey, United States, 1971-1973.* Hyattsville, MD. Vital & Health Statistics, 1(10a).

NCHS, 1975. *Data Evaluations and Research Methods: Distribution of Variance and Properties Estimators for Complex Multistage Probability Samples An Empirical Distribution.* Hyattsville, MD. Vital & Health Statistics 2(65).

NCHS, 1977. *Plan and Operation of the Health and Nutrition Examination Survey, United States, 1971-1973.* Hyattsville, MD. Vital & Health Statistics 1(10b).

NCHS, 1978. *Plan and Operation of the NHANES I Augmentation Survey of Adults 25-74 Years, United States, 1974-1975.* Hyattsville, MD. Vital & Health Statistics 1(14).

NCHS, 1981. *Plan and Operation of the Second National Health and Nutrition Examination Survey, 1976–80.* Hyattsville, MD. Vital & Health Statistics 1(15).

NCHS, 1982. *A Statistical Methodology for Analyzing Data from a Complex Survey: The First National Health and Nutrition Examination Survey.* Hyattsville, MD. Vital & Health Statistics 2(92).

NCHS, 1985. *Plan and Operation of the Hispanic Health and Nutrition Examination Survey 1982-1984.* Hyattsville, MD. Vital & Health Statistics 1(19).

NCHS, 1987. *Plan and Operation of the NHANES I Epidemiologic Followup Study, 1982-84.* Hyattsville, MD. Vital & Health Statistics 1(22).

NCHS, 1990. *Plan and Operation of the NHANES I Epidemiologic Followup Study, 1986.* Hyattsville, MD. Vital & Health Statistics 1(25).

NCHS, 1992a. *Plan and Operation of the NHANES I Epidemiologic Followup Study, 1987.* Hyattsville, MD. Vital & Health Statistics 1(27).

NCHS, 1992b. *Sample Design: Third National Health and Nutrition Examination Survey.* Hyattsville, MD. Vital and Health Statistics 2(113).

NCHS, 1994a. *National Health and Nutrition Examination Survey III: Accounting for Item Nonresponse Bias.* Hyattsville, MD.

NCHS, 1994b. *Plan and Operation of the Third National Health and Nutrition Examination Survey*, 1988–94. Hyattsville, MD. Vital Health Statistics 1(32).

NCHS, 1996a. *Analytic and Reporting Guidelines: Third National Health and Nutrition Examination Survey, 1988-94.* Hyattsville, MD.

NCHS, 1996b. *Analytic and Reporting Guidelines: Third National Health and Nutrition Examination Survey, 1988-94. Appendix B.* Hyattsville, MD.

NCHS, 1996c. *National Health and Nutrition Examination Survey III, Weighting and Estimation Methodology, Executive Summary.* Hyattsville, MD. <http://www.cdc.gov/nchs/about/major/nhanes/nhanes3/cdrom/NCHS/MANUALS/WGT_EXEC.PDF>.

NCHS, 1996d. *The National Health and Nutrition Examination Surveys, A Selective Bibliography, 1980-96.* October. This information was distributed on floppy discs to NHANES Consortium members by NCHS.

NCHS, 1997. *Plan and Operation of the NHANES I Epidemiologic Followup Study, 1992.* Hyattsville, MD. Vital & Health Statistics 1(35).

NCHS, 1999a. *Plan and Operation of the NHANES II Mortality Study, 1992.* Hyattsville, MD. Vital & Health Statistics 1(38).

NCHS, 1999b. *NHANES- A Selective Bibliography 1997-1999.* Hyattsville, MD. <http://www.cdc.gov/nchs/about/major/nhanes/97-99jan00.pdf>.

NCHS, 2001. *Laboratory Procedures Manual.* April. Hyattsville, MD. <http://www.cdc.gov/nchs/about/major/nhanes/lab7-11.pdf>.

NCHS, 2001a. *MEC Interviewers Procedures Manual.* Revised January. Hyattsville, MD. <http://www.cdc.gov/nchs/about/major/nhanes/c1-4_int.pdf>.

NCHS, 2001b. *MEC Interviewers Procedures Manual, Part IV.* Hyattsville, MD. <http://www.cdc.gov/nchs/about/major/nhanes/int4.pdf>.

U.S. EPA (U.S. Environmental Protection Agency), 1986. *Air Quality Criteria for Lead.* Research Triangle Park, North Carolina:, Office of Health and Environmental Assessment; EPA report no. EPA-600/8-83/028aF-dF.

U.S.DHHS (U.S. Department of Health and Human Services), 1988. *The nature and extent of lead poisoning in children in the United States: a report to Congress.* Public Health Service, Agency for Toxic Substances and Disease Registry. Atlanta.